A Pocket Guide for Student Midwives

A Pocket Guide for Student Midwives

Stella McKay-Moffat

MPhil., BA (Hons) RN, RM, ADM, Cert. Ed.
Family Planning Certificate
Senior Lecturer Midwifery, Edge Hill College

Pam Lee

MA (Social policy), BA (Hons) RN, RM, MTD, Dip. N (Lond.) FETC
Dip. Applied Social Sciences, ENB NO7
Post Grad. Diploma in Psycho-sexual therapy
Senior Lecturer Midwifery, Edge Hill College

John Wiley & Sons, Ltd

Copyright © 2006   John Wiley & Sons, Ltd, The Atrium, Southern Gate, Chichester, West
                    Sussex PO19 8SQ, England
                    Telephone (+44) 1243 779777

Email (for orders and customer service enquiries): cs-books@wiley.co.uk
Visit our Home Page on www.wiley.com

Other Wiley Editorial Offices

John Wiley & Sons Inc., 111 River Street, Hoboken, NJ 07030, USA

Jossey-Bass, 989 Market Street, San Francisco, CA 94103-1741, USA

Wiley-VCH Verlag GmbH, Boschstr. 12, D-69469 Weinheim, Germany

John Wiley & Sons Australia Ltd, 42 McDougall Street, Milton, Queensland 4064, Australia

John Wiley & Sons (Asia) Pte Ltd, 2 Clementi Loop #02-01, Jin Xing Distripark, Singapore
129809

John Wiley & Sons Canada Ltd, 22 Worcester Road, Etobicoke, Ontario, Canada M9W 1L1

Wiley also publishes its books in a variety of electronic formats. Some content that appears in
print may not be available in electronic books.

Library of Congress Cataloging-in-Publication Data

McKay-Moffat, Stella.
    A pocket guide for student midwives / Stella McKay-Moffat, Pamela Lee.
       p.   ;   cm.
    Includes bibliographical references and index.
    ISBN 0-470-01978-6 (pbk. : alk. paper)
 1. Midwifery – Handbooks, manuals, etc.
    [DNLM: 1. Midwifery – Handbooks.   WQ 165 M478p 2006]   I. Lee, Pamela, RN.
 II. Title.
    RG950.M43 2006
    618.2 – dc22
                                                                    2006005573

British Library Cataloguing in Publication Data

A catalogue record for this book is available from the British Library

ISBN-13 978-0-470-01978-8 (pbk)
ISBN-10 0-470-01978-6 (pbk)

Typeset in Photina MT 9.5/13 by SNP Best-set Typesetter Ltd., Hong Kong
Printed and bound in Great Britain by TJ International, Padstow

This book is printed on acid-free paper responsibly manufactured from sustainable forestry in
which at least two trees are planted for each one used for paper production.

This book is dedicated to all our student midwives, past, present and future, who not only 'keep us on our toes' by providing us with challenges, but teach us, and reward us with their success

Contents

		Page
About the authors		ix
Foreword, by Dame Lorna Muirhead, DBE, President of the Royal College of Midwives 1997–2004		x
Preface		xi

Section 1 **The Language of Midwifery**
Terms, abbreviations, definitions   1

Section 2 **Quick Reference Topics**
Conditions, procedures, emergency situations, supporting information, e.g. voluntary organisations   20

Figures	**Flow / action charts**	
1	Antepartum haemorrhage	31
2	Neonatal resuscitation	38
3.1	Cord prolapse – presentation at home	70
3.2	Cord prolapse – presentation in hospital	71
4	Apgar score	80
5.1	Management of third stage of labour – physiological and active	82
5.2	Management of third stage of labour – alternative active management	83
6	Disseminated intravascular coagulation (DIC)	95
7	Eclampsia	97

8	Genetic inheritance, e.g. PKU	163
9	Post-partum haemorrhage – primary	178
10	Post-partum haemorrhage – secondary	179
11.1	Retained placenta – at home	202
11.2	Retained placenta – in hospital	203
12	Shoulder dystocia	208
13	Uterine inversion	229
14	Uterine rupture	231

Diagrams

1.1, 1.2, 1.3	Delivery of occipito-posterior position	84–85
2.1, 2.2, 2.3	Delivery of face presentation	86–87
3.1	Normal haemoglobin composition	110
3.2.1, 3.2.2	Normal adult haemoglobins	110
3.3	Normal fetal haemoglobin	110
3.4.1, 3.4.2	Sickle cell haemoglobins	111
3.5.1, 3.5.2	Alpha thalassaemia	113
3.6.1, 3.6.2	Beta thalassaemia	114
4	Heel prick sites	118
5.1 to 5.9	Placenta types	166–170
6	Stations of the head in the pelvis	233

References   237

About the authors

Stella and Pam are very experienced midwives and midwifery lecturers having taught a range of learners from pre-registration students to qualified staff. Both authors embrace innovation and advancement in the maternity services and midwifery profession, whilst valuing the quality of appropriate traditional practices.

Stella spent over fifteen years in practice, with more than eleven of those in the community offering the whole range of maternity services, including home birth. She has a keen interest in women's health, and in particular in contraception and family planning. Her Mphil. research explored maternity services for women with disabilities and midwives' experiences of providing those services.

Having gained an MA in Social Policy, Pam has a special interest in the social policy-making process, particularly in relation to the maternity services. Another area of her interest and expertise is around sexuality and body image, and Pam is a qualified Psychosexual Therapist within the Women's Sexual Health services of a local trust. Pam acts as an external examiner for Anglia Poly University (APU) on the Human Sexuality and Midwifery programme.

Foreword

When entering the world of midwifery it is necessary to know the language used, and to understand exactly what that language means so that midwives can be confident, and so that practice can be safe. This itself is a great challenge along with everything else there is to learn, which is why this instant reference book, that can accompany you wherever you work, is timely.

I have thoroughly enjoyed reading *A Pocket Guide for Student Midwives*, and indeed I have learned from it. How I wish it had been in my pocket when I was a new midwife, and for that matter when I was mature in the profession! Instant reference to it could have saved me the anxieties we all face from time to time, sometimes when everyone else is busy and has little time to reassure us, and especially when things go wrong and action needs to be taken quickly.

All midwives will find a wealth of information within the pages of this book, which I enthusiastically recommend, and wish it, and you, every success.

Dame Lorna Muirhead, DBE
President of the Royal College of Midwives 1997–2004

Preface

This book was inspired by comments from the student midwives in the authors' educational institution. They said, 'We need something to help us survive the midwifery course.' Both authors are aware of students' anxieties and frustration at the vast amount of information and skills that have to be learned to become a midwife.

Midwifery is a practice-based profession that is both an art and a science. However, there are frequently many different ways of achieving the same satisfactory learning outcome: the lack of 'black and white' or 'hard and fast' rules in the majority of the elements of the profession may make learning difficult to cope with. This is particularly noticeable as practitioners are striving, in line with the philosophy of *Changing Childbirth* (DoH 1993), to facilitate choice and control for women and their partners. Nevertheless, once the 'basics' of a situation have been learnt, the 'variations' can be added to the repertoire of knowledge and skills.

Practice needs to be underpinned by a sound theoretical framework that is evidence-based. In an endeavour to help students grasp the appropriate knowledge and understanding, link theory to practice and 'survive the midwifery course', the following pocket book has been written to provide quick, easy-to-read information and guidelines on the 'basics' in midwifery that could be taken on duty. The instant access to information will provide some theory, trigger thought and give directions to support practice in an easily repeatable process.

This book is written with both degree and diploma student midwives in mind. Those students previously registered nurses may find that some of the basic nursing procedures are already within their capabilities. Nevertheless, revision is often useful, and some procedures may, in fact, have a different focus, as they are centred on the (generally) healthy childbearing woman rather than the sick patient.

The book is in two sections, each alphabetical. The first section contains some of the language of midwifery: terms, abbreviations and definitions. A few terms are colloquial and not necessarily 'medically' correct, but are included, however, to enable clarification of understanding and to prompt the use of correct terminology. The second section contains common conditions, procedures, emergency situations, and supporting information. Where conditions are noted the aetiology is given, if known. Each topic may include further factors that involve recognition, prevention, and actions to take in an emergency situation that may be in the form of flow/action charts. These action charts should be read from top left. The flow lines are followed depending on the circumstances at the time. The procedures that are included have an overview of the 'how to' (frequently including the preparation needed); and the 'why', supported by research or evidence, and Midwives' rules and standards (Nurses and Midwives Council (NMC) 2004b) and The NMC code of professional conduct: standards for conduct, performance and ethics (NMC 2004a). The references used could provide useful evidence to support practice. Finally, the supporting information is varied, and ranges from details about Government and international initiatives to available support groups and useful websites.

As no topic is in isolation, many categories are cross-referenced and extra reading / activities are suggested to enhance the reader's knowledge. Furthermore, additional study may be needed to understand and learn the anatomy, the physiology, and possibly the biochemistry associated with the conditions included. Finally, the authors appreciate that local policies and protocols vary; therefore the reader is recommended to consider topics in the light of those local guidelines as well as of the emergence of new evidence that informs practice.

Acknowledgements

We would like to thank Lawrence Berry, Media Resources Officer at Edge Hill College, for his help and expertise in producing the graphics, and Carol Revill-Johnson, Midwifery Lecturer / Practitioner and Advanced Life Support in Obstetrics trainer, for her constructive criticism of the action flow charts.

The Language of Midwifery

1

In a new environment one key to understanding is to have the knowledge of the language that is used. To this end, this section contains an alphabetical list of terms, abbreviations and definitions frequently used in midwifery, nursing and medicine. Terms in italics may be heard but are colloquial; however, they are included here to help understanding of the 'everyday' language used, but also to encourage the use of correct terminology.

Symbols are frequently used as a 'shorthand'; therefore some commonly used ones are included at the beginning of this section of the book.

$\cong$ approximate	$\leq$ less than or equal to
$\geq$ more than or equal to	Δ diagnosis
$\uparrow$ raised / increased	$\downarrow$ lowered / decreased
$<$ less than / before	$>$ greater than / after
R_x prescribe / prescription	# fracture(d) (usually bone)
? query, question, possible	μmol/l micromol per litre

ABO blood groups – classification system according to the presence of antigens on red blood cells / antibodies in serum (see also **Rhesus factor**)

blood group	antigen on cell	antibody in serum
O	none	anti A and anti B
A	A	anti B
B	B	anti A
AB	A and B	none

blood group O Rh negative = universal donor (can give to any group in an emergency)

blood group AB Rh positive = universal recipient (can receive from any group in an emergency)

Abortion – expulsion of the products of conception from the uterus <24th week of gestation – can be induced (termination) or spontaneous (miscarriage)

Acceleration / active phase of cervical dilatation – more rapid cervical dilation after 5 cm – recorded on a partogram (approx. 1 cm per hour)

Acceleration / augmentation of labour – process by which spontaneous labour is made more efficient through intervention

Accountability – liablity to be called to account for one's conduct, responsibility for practising professionally

Active birth – one in which the woman participates fully in her labour, is fully aware of what is going on in her body and is able to respond naturally

Active management of labour – assessing / monitoring progress and implementing policies to prevent prolonged labour (see **acceleration / augmentation of labour**)

Adoption – a formal legal procedure that severs the relationship between a child and its parent(s) and establishes a new one with its adoptive parents.

Adoption Agency/Society – a local authority (LA) or voluntary organisation whose function consists of or includes making arrangements for the adoption of children. Voluntary agencies must be registered with the LA and open to inspection, and are non-profit-making, but may charge fees for services provided.

AFP – alpha fetoprotein – a precursor to plasma protein produced by the fetus and excreted into the amniotic fluid. High levels of AFP in maternal blood can be used as part of a risk assessment for fetal neural tube defects and low levels for the risk of Down's syndrome. Prenatal diagnosis of neural tube defects is effected by assessing AFP in the liquor following amniocentesis.

Alternative birth positions – positions other than the dorsal position that the mother may choose when giving birth, e.g. a squatting position, an upright position

Amnion – a tough, smooth, translucent membrane derived from the inner cell mass of the embryo. It lines the chorion and the fetal surface of the placenta as far as the insertion of the umbilical cord. It contains the amniotic fluid (liquor) and contributes to its formation

Amniotomy – rupturing the forewaters – see **ARM, acceleration / augmentation of labour**

AN – antenatal(ly)

Anaesthesia – loss of sensation induced by anaesthetic agents to allow surgery – total anaesthesia / partial anaesthesia, with / without loss of consciousness.

Analgesia – insensibility to pain without loss of consciousness, pain relief.

Antepartum haemorrhage (APH) – bleeding from the genital tract >24 weeks of pregnancy

Anti D immunoglobulin – a blood product given IM to Rhesus-negative women to prevent isoimmunisation to the D part of the Rhesus factor (see **Rhesus factor**, and Wray and Jackson-Baker 2000)

Apgar Score – a scoring system devised by Dr Virginia Apgar in 1958 to assess the newborn's condition for resuscitation purposes (see Figure 4)

APH (Antepartum haemorrhage) – bleeding from the genital tract >24 weeks of pregnancy

APTT – activated partial thromboplastin time – a blood test related to the clotting mechanism

ARDS – adult / acute respiratory distress syndrome (see **RDS**)

ARM – artificial rupture of membranes, i.e. manually perforating the bag of forewaters containing the fetus (see also Section 2 and **acceleration / augmentation of labour**)

AST – aspartate aminotransferase – an enzyme that catalyses salts of the amino acid aspartamine – blood levels raised with liver / heart damaged (see **PIH** and **pre-eclampsia** in Sections 1 and 2)

Attitude – relationship of fetal head and limbs to the trunk, e.g. flexion, deflexion, (military attitude) partial extension and full extension

Baby – the fetus when completely expelled from the uterus >24 weeks gestation.

Baby blues – 3rd / 4th day blues – feeling emotionally low following childbirth (see **postnatal depression** in Section 2)

Bandl's ring – an exaggerated retraction ring that occurs when labour is obstructed – ? palpated abdominally, and is a serious sign (see **retraction ring**)

Barlow's test – screening test for CDH, modified from Ortolani's test

Battledore insertion – cord inserted at the very edge of the placenta (see Diagram 5.4)

BBA – born before arrival, i.e. baby born before arrival of midwife / doctor

BD – twice daily – often on a prescription

BF – Breastfeeding

BFI – Breast Feeding Initiative (see Section 2)

Biophysical profile – assessment of the fetal condition using indicators such as fetal breathing movements, doppler techniques, amniotic fluid measurement

Bipartite / tripartite placenta – one divided into two or three distinct areas (see Diagram 5.9)

Bishop's score – method of assessing the suitability of the cervix for induction of labour by noting the length and softness and dilatation of the cervical os (opening)

Blades – obstetric forceps

BM sticks / test – originally a colour-changing reagent strip for measuring peripheral blood glucose made by Boehringer Mannheim. Term often used colloquially for all estimations of peripheral blood glucose. Modern sticks from various makers are used with an electrical optical measuring device for greater accuracy.

BO – bowels opened, i.e. faeces passed

Bradycardia – slowing of the heart rate, in adults <60 beats per minute, in the fetus <100 beats per minute.

Brandt–Andrews – method of delivering the placenta without oxytocic drugs (see **delivery technique** – third stage flow chart in Section 2)

Braxton Hicks contractions – painless uterine contractions, part of the physiological growth / stretching process during pregnancy.

Breech – the lower fetal pole, including buttocks and legs (see **presentation**; and **breech delivery** in Section 2)

Brim of the pelvis – bony ring formed by the following landmarks (posteriorly to anteriorly): sacral promontory, sacral ala or wing, sacro-iliac joint, iliopectineal line, iliopectineal eminence, superior ramus of the pubic bone, upper inner body of the pubic bone and the symphysis pubis, continuing round in a circle

Brow – area on fetal skull from supra-orbital ridges to coronal suture (see **presentation**; and **occipito-posterior position** in Section 2)

Buttonholing – of perineum, i.e. as the perineum is distending during advancement of the fetal head, small areas of tissue begin to separate, causing an opening

C & S – request on a form sent to laboratory with a specimen, e.g. MSSU, HVS – for culture (growth and identification of the organism) and testing its sensitivity (to antibiotics that may be used against it)

Caput succedaneum – soft swelling of fluid (oedema) on the fetal scalp due to pressure on the head during labour (can cross a suture line of the skull bones – compare with cephalhaematoma)

CCT – controlled cord traction (see **delivery technique**, third-stage management in Section 2)

CDH – congenital dislocation of the hip

CEMACH – Confidential Enquiry into Maternal and Child Health (see Section 2)

CEMD – Confidential Enquiry into Maternal Deaths (see Section 2)

Ceph – cephalic = pertaining to the fetal head

Cephalhaematoma – swelling on newborn's head due to bleeding beneath the periosteum associated with traumatic delivery (does not cross a suture line of the skull – compare with caput succedaneum)

Cephalic – pertaining to the fetal head (see **presentation**)

Cephalo-pelvic disproportion (CPD) – fetal head will not pass through the maternal pelvis (see Section 2)

Cervix – the lower one-third of the uterus

CESDI – Confidential Enquiry into Stillbirth and Deaths in Infancy (see Section 2)

Chasing the dragon – smoking heroin (diamorphine) by lighting the powder on aluminium foil and inhaling the fumes

Chignon – swelling on newborn's head following vacuum extraction (see **instrumental delivery** in Section 2) as soft tissues are drawn into the cup during the procedure (see **caput succedaneum**)

Chorion – a thick, opaque, friable membrane that develops from the trophoblast. It is continuous with the edge of the placenta and is closely adherent to the decidua

CIN – cervical intra-epithelial neoplasm – early cervical cell changes that could progress to cancer if not treated

Circumvallate placenta – one with a double fold of chorion round the edge of the placenta, causing a ridge (see Diagrams 5.7, 5.8)

CONI – care of next infant (see **sudden infant death syndrome** in Section 2)

Confidentiality – a trusting relationship in which secrets may be imparted – the midwife has a duty to respect confidentiality except where disclosure is required by law (see NMC 2004a *The Code of Professional Conduct: Standards for Conduct, Performance and Ethics*)

Coombs test – performed on cord blood to detect maternal antibodies on fetal red cells (see **Rhesus factor**)

Cotyledon – a clump of chorionic villi surrounded by maternal blood: 10–30 of them form the maternal surface of the placenta, i.e. the surface attached to the uterus (see Diagram 5.1)

CPD – cephalo-pelvic disproportion (see **prolonged labour** in Sections 1 and 2)

CPR – cardiopulmonary resuscitation

Cracking on – labour is progressing, often rapidly

Crash bleep – emergency bleep – method of urgently summoning aid (usually medical) – familiarise yourself with your unit's protocol

Cricoid pressure – occlusion of the oesophagus by pressure applied to the cricoid cartilage (i.e. Sellick's manoeuvre) to prevent inhalation of reflux of stomach content during initiation of anaesthetic and before an endotracheal tube (ET) is inserted to maintain the airway

CSF – cerebro-spinal fluid

CT / CAT scan – computerised (computer-assisted) tomography, i.e. computers record body 'slices' from X-ray scan pictures

CTG – cardiotocograph

Curve of Carus – an arc from the pelvic brim to the pelvic outlet, i.e. through the true pelvis, which the baby passes through during labour and birth

CVP – central venous pressure, i.e. right atrium blood pressure – indicates circulatory function / blood volume, especially in shock / during blood replacement

Denominator – a fixed point on the presenting part determining the fetal position

Diabetes mellitus – a disorder of carbohydrate metabolism – insufficient insulin production / inability of cell response to insulin resulting in high blood glucose levels – may occur in pregnancy without any previous history (gestational diabetes)

Diameter – a measurement from one point to another through the pelvis or the fetal skull

DIC – **disseminated intravascular coagulation** (coagulopathy) – specific conditions result in excessive use of clotting factors, leading to bleeding that is difficult to control

Dips – falls in fetal heart rate – correct terminology = decelerations

Directed pushing – instructing the mother to bear down with each contraction (see **Valsalva manoeuvre**)

Dizygotic – developing from two ova and sperms (see **multiple pregnancy** in Sections 1 and 2)

DTA – **deep transverse arrest**, i.e. the baby's head has become lodged in the pelvis in the transverse diameter, needing rotation with forceps or delivery by caesarean section

Dubowitz Score – system for assessing baby's gestational age using neurological and physical criteria

DVT – **deep vein thrombosis** (blood clot), commonly found in a calf vein

Eclampsia – serious pregnancy complication where eclamptic convulsions occur – usually follows fulminating pre-eclampsia, possibly without previous signs / symptoms, especially postnatally

ECV – **external cephalic version**

EDD / EDC – **estimated / expected date of delivery / confinement**: calculated by adding 7 days and 9 months to first day (of bleeding) of last menstrual period (LMP) = Naegele's rule: accuracy challenged – see Olsen (1999)

Edinburgh postnatal depression score – a questionnaire designed to help predict which women are at risk of postnatal depression

Embryo – the developing conceptus from the third to the eighth week following fertilisation

Engagement of the fetal head – when the widest part of the head passes through the pelvic brim (usually the biparietal diameter)

Epidural block – a method of giving analgesia / anaesthesia by putting a local anaesthetic agent into the epidural space

Ergometrine – an oxytocic agent with a sustained uterine action – takes 6–7 minutes to act when given IM (0.5 mg) – can also be given IV – acts within 45 seconds (0.25 mg)

ESR – erythrocyte sedimentation rate: measures the distance (in millimetres) that red blood cells settle in unclotted blood toward the bottom of a specially marked test tube over the course of an hour. Useful in detecting and monitoring infection, including tuberculosis, tissue necrosis and rheumatism and arthritis.

ET tube – endotracheal tube – tube passed into trachea to maintain an open airway; has an outer cuff that is inflated with air to make a seal

Face – area on fetal skull from where the head joins the neck to the coronal suture and anterior fontanelle (see **presentation**; and **delivery technique** in Section 2)

Fallot's tetralogy – cardiac abnormality causing cyanotic heart disease: comprises pulmonary stenosis, overriding aorta, ventricular septal defect and right ventricular hypertrophy

FBC – full blood count, i.e. numbers of all types of cells – often on a laboratory request form

Fetal distress – the fetus suffers oxygen deprivation and becomes hypoxic (see **birth asphyxia** in Section 2)

Fetus – the developing conceptus from the end of the eighth week until birth, when it becomes a neonate

FH, FHH or FHHR – fetal heart, fetal heart heard / heard and regular

First degree tear – involves the vaginal mucosa and / or the skin of the perineum, but not muscle

Flat baby (not an acceptable term) – asphyxiated baby (see **birth asphyxia** in Section 2)

FM / FMF – fetal movements / movements felt

Folic acid – a member of the vitamin B complex occurring in green plants, fresh fruit, liver and yeast – necessary for normal fetal CNS development – advised as a supplement pre-conception and in early pregnancy (see **neural tube defect** in Section 2)

Fontanelle – membranous space on baby's skull where two or more suture lines meet (see **vaginal examination** in Section 2)

Forewaters – amniotic fluid trapped before the fetal head as labour progresses (see **ARM** and **vaginal examination** in Section 2)

Fourchette – a fold of skin between the vaginal entrance and the perineum

FSE – fetal scalp electrode – for continuous electronic monitoring of FH (see **CTG**)

Full dilatation of the cervix – when no cervix is felt on vaginal examination – 10 cm

Fundus – upper part of the uterus between the areas of fallopian tube insertion (the cornua)

GA – **general anaesthetic**

Gas and air – gaseous mixture of 50% oxygen / 50% nitrous oxide (Entonox) inhaled for analgesia during labour

Gas man – nickname for an anaesthetist

Gestation – period during embryonic growth from conception to birth – hence, gestational age; but pregnancy is counted from the first day of the last menstrual period (LMP) – it is not always clear which calculation is being used

Glabella – the bridge of the nose; glabellar tap – primitive reflex elicited in the newborn (see **initial newborn examination** in Section 2)

Gown up – dressing in a sterile gown (frequently green) – prior to aseptic / sterile technique, ensuring gown sterility is not broken

Gravid – pregnant; hence gravidity (number of times pregnant), primigravida, multigravida

Guthrie test – phenylketonuria screening 8–10 days following birth – microbiological techniques are used on filter paper soaked with blood – seldom used now (see also **Scriver test**; and **heel prick** in Section 2)

Haemorrhoids – varicose veins of the rectum / anus common in pregnancy owing to the effects of progesterone (see **varicose veins** in Section 2)

Haemorrhage – excessive blood loss leading to shock (see **antepartum** and **post-partum haemorrhage** in Sections 1 and 2)

Hb – **haemoglobin** – blood levels routinely screened for (see **anaemia** in Section 2)

HV – **Health Visitor**

HVS – **high vaginal swab** – infection screening

Hydatidiform mole – gestational trophoblastic disease, usually without development of the fetus

Hypertension – abnormally high arterial blood pressure, a diastolic blood pressure of 90 mmHg significantly high in pregnancy (see **pregnancy-induced hypertension and pre-eclampsia** in Section 2)

Hypoglycaemia – reduction in blood glucose levels; normal fasting blood glucose = 3–5 mmol/l (adult), less in the neonate (see **heel prick** in Section 2)

Hypothermia – reduction in body temperature, below 36°C in the neonate

ICU – **intensive care unit**

IDD / IDDM – **insulin-dependent diabetes / insulin-dependent diabetes mellitus**

IM – **intramuscular** – an injection into a muscle (see **administration of drugs** in Section 2)

Induction of labour – initiation of labour by artificial means

Infant – baby from birth to the end of the first year.

INR – international normalised ratio – a blood test measuring the ratios of clotting factors as part the clotting mechanism screening

Insulin – hormone produced by the islets of Langerhans in the pancreas – a transport mechanism for glucose / regulates carbohydrate metabolism; given synthetically in diabetes mellitus

Intrapartum – during birth (second stage of labour)

Intrauterine growth retardation (IUGR) – fetal growth falling below that expected, when the birth weight is below the tenth centile for gestational age (see **intrauterine growth retardation** and **small for gestational age babies** in Section 2)

Intubation – passage of an endotracheal (ET) tube into the trachea for resuscitation purposes and to maintain a clear airway

Involution of the uterus – the process by which the uterus shrinks to its pre-pregnant shape, size, and situation – brought about by autolysis and phagocytosis

IUCD / IUD – intrauterine contraceptive device (coil) – beware of next abbreviation

IUD – intrauterine death (note abbreviation above)

IUGR – intrauterine growth retardation

IV – intravenous: usually an injection / infusion (see **administration of drugs** in Section 2)

IVI – intravenous infusion

Jaundice – yellow skin / mucous membranes discoloration when serum bilirubin levels reach 80 μmol/l

Karyotype – a visual arrangement of all chromosomes from a single cell, enabling identification / counting

Kernicterus – staining of the basal ganglia in the brain due to high levels of unconjugated (fat-soluble) bilirubin – causes severe damage, including blindness, deafness and cerebral palsy (see **jaundice** in Section 2)

Ketoacidosis – metabolic disorder resulting from insufficient carbohydrate intake; fats are metabolised instead, and ketone bodies formed (see **diabetes mellitus**)

Kleihauer test – blood test on Rhesus-negative women estimating the number of fetal blood cells in maternal circulation following delivery – large numbers ? extra anti-D immunoglobulin

Labour – a continuous physiological process of contraction and retraction (shortening) of the myometrium (uterine muscle) during which the products of conception are expelled from the uterus.

1. First stage – sometimes considered to be in three phases, although demarcation is imprecise and there is no professional consensus
   Latent phase: (equates to the lay definition of 'slow labour') the early preparation stage, lasting hours or days. Contractions may be regular or irregular, frequent or intermittent, painful or painless, weak or fairly strong. The cervix slowly dilates from closed (in primigravida) or slightly open, i.e. multips os (in multigravida), up to approximately 4 cm dilated.
   Active or acceleration phase – a continuation of the latent phase, i.e. established labour. Contractions become progressively more regular, frequent, strong and painful. Cervical dilatation progresses at approximately 1 cm per hour to full dilatation (about 10 cm), and the presenting part (the fetal head in normal labour) progresses through the maternal pelvis.
   Deceleration phase – progress of cervical dilatation from 9 cm to 10 cm is sometimes delayed as contractions briefly fade (mother and uterus 'rest') before full dilatation is achieved – causes no concern unless there is fetal distress.
2. Second stage – from full dilatation of the cervix to expulsion of the baby. The mother may not immediately have the urge to bear down (push) – await spontaneous expulsive effort (pushing), which is less traumatic for mother and baby than directed pushing (see **Valsalva manoeuvre** below) unless there are signs of fetal distress – some mothers do need guidance and encouragement.
3. Third stage – from the birth of the baby until complete expulsion of placenta and membranes and the control of haemorrhage.

Lanugo – fine, down-like hair on the fetal body – some often remains at birth
Last menstrual period (LMP) – the first day of bleeding in a normal menstrual cycle; used to calculate the expected date of delivery (EDD)
Latent phase of cervical dilatation – slow dilatation of the cervix up to 5 cm, seen especially in the primigravida; recorded on the partogram
Lecithin/sphingomyelin (LS) ratio – a test performed on amniotic fluid to determine fetal lung maturity – should be greater than 2:1 (see **antenatal screening** in Section 2)
Lie – the relationship of the long axis of the fetus (fetal spine) to the long axis of the mother's uterus – usually longitudinal – ? oblique, transverse, unstable (see **abdominal palpation** in Section 2)
Live birth – any baby born who breathes, cries or shows signs of life
LMP – Last menstrual period – the first day of bleeding in a normal menstrual cycle, used to calculate the expected date of delivery (EDD)
Lochia – the discharges from the uterus following delivery – may be rubra, serosa or albicans

LS ratio – the lecithin–sphingomyelin ratio in amniotic fluid, normally 2 : 1, used as an indicator of lung surfactant levels and therefore lung maturity. A lower ratio indicates the potential for neonatal respiratory distress syndrome.

Malposition – where the occiput is posterior in the pelvis rather than the normal anterior

Malpresentation – where the fetal part lying lowest in the birth canal is not the normal vertex – i.e. face, brow, shoulder, breech, or compound presentation, such as e.g. head and hand

Matthews Duncan – method of placental separation – the placenta is lying in the lower uterus and 'slides' off the wall – the maternal surface of the placenta appears at the vulva – often associated with excessive blood loss (the so-called *dirty Duncan*); compare with the Schultz method

MCH – mean corpuscular haemoglobin (reported on blood test) – average amount of haemoglobin in the red blood cells (see **anaemia** in Section 2)

MCV – mean corpuscular volume (reported on blood test) – average volume of a single red blood cell in cubic micrometers (μm), normally 90 (see **anaemia** in Section 2)

Mechanism of labour – means by which the fetus negotiates the birth canal

Meconium (mec.) – greenish-black substance present in fetal intestine / passed during the first 2–3 days of life – fresh / old meconium in liquor indicates how recently passed (see **fetal distress**)

Mentum – chin – the denominator in a face presentation (see **presentation**)

Monozygotic – developing from one ovum and sperm (see **dizygotic** and **multiple pregnancy**)

Morbidity – state of ill health / disease; case numbers of a particular disease in a given population – commonly related to maternal / perinatal mortality

Mortality – death, the frequency / number of deaths in a given population – commonly related to maternal or perinatal morbidity – (see **Confidential Enquiry into Maternal Deaths (CEMD)**, **Confidential Enquiry into Maternal and Child Health (CEMACH)**, **Confidential Enquiry into Sudden Deaths in Infancy (CESDI)** in Section 2)

Moulding – the alteration in shape of fetal skull allowing passage through the true pelvis – engaging diameter is reduced at the expense of the diameter at 90° to it

MRI scan – magnetic resonance imaging scan – computers used to map variations in body tissue subjected to high-frequency radio waves – particularly useful for examining the central nervous system

MSSU – midstream specimen of urine (see **UTI**)

Multigravida – a woman pregnant for the second or subsequent time (even if the previous pregnancy/ies resulted in miscarriage) – a grand(e) multigravida is a woman pregnant for a fifth or subsequent time

Multips' os – the state of cervical os (opening), often used to mean the cervix itself: i.e. it is not showing any indications that the woman is in labour, only that she has previously had a baby

Multiple pregnancy – simultaneous presence of more then one fetus

NAD – **nothing abnormal discovered** – commonly referring to results of a standard dip stick urine test, ? other examinations

NCT – **National Childbirth Trust**

Neonatal / neonate – the period from birth / baby up until 28 days

Niggler – a woman in spurious labour, i.e. having contractions but not in established labour

NNU / NNICU – **neonatal unit / neonatal intensive care unit**

Nocte – at night – often on a prescription

NTD – **neural tube defect**, e.g. spina bifida

OA – **occipito-anterior**, i.e. the occiput (back of fetal head) is in the anterior part of the maternal pelvis; direct OA = behind symphysis pubis; LOA or ROA = to left or right of symphysis pubis

Obs. or doing the Obs., i.e. observations – noting vital signs, e.g. temperature, pulse, blood pressure, respirations, ? others – e.g. fluid balance, level of consciousness

Obstetric forceps – two-bladed stainless steel instruments (see **instrumental delivery** in Section 2)

Obstructed labour – no advance of presenting part despite good uterine contractions (see **prolonged labour**)

Occiput – occipital bone of fetal skull – denominator in vertex presentation (see **presentation**)

ODP / ODA / ODO – **operating department practitioner /assistant / orderly** – assists the anaesthetist

OES – **obstetric emergency service** / *flying squad* – less frequently deployed for community obstetric emergencies as paramedics become more skilled / available

OP position – **occipito-posterior position**, i.e. fetal occiput (back of head) in posterior part of maternal pelvis; direct OP = occiput in mother's sacrum; LOP, ROP = left or right of sacrum

Ophthalmia neonatorum – purulent eye discharge of the newborn occurring within 21 days of birth – no longer a notifiable disease – ? caused by *Gonococcus* organism / *Chlamydia trachomatis*

Ortolani's test – screening method for congenital dislocation of the hip, modified by Barlow

Oxytocic drugs – synthetic drugs mimicking the action of oxytocin from the posterior pituitary gland and causing uterine contractions (ergometrine, Syntometrine, Syntocinon)

Paed. – short for paediatrician

Parity – number of pregnancies >24 weeks, hence para 1, 2, multipara, grand(e) multipara (>4 babies)

Partogram / partograph – a chart for graphically entering salient features of labour – progress represented visually, allowing easy recognition of deviations from normal

Parturition – childbirth; parity

Pelvimetry – accurate measurement of true pelvis performed by X-ray, carried out if cephalo-pelvic disproportion (CPD) is suspected

Perinatal – period before birth, at birth and up to one week following birth

PET = Pre-eclamptic toxaemia – no longer an accepted term (see **PIH / pre-eclampsia**)

PIH – pregnancy-induced hypertension

PIPPIN – Parents in Partnership Parent Infant Network – a national charity whose aim is to improve the emotional health of families at the time surrounding the birth of a baby; they also offer training courses for professionals (see Section 2)

PKU – phenylketonuria – inborn error of metabolism (see Section 2)

PN – postnatal(ly)

Position – relationship of denominator to a fixed point on the pelvis, e.g. right occipito-anterior (ROA) (see **abdominal palpation** in Section 2)

Postmaturity / post-term – pregnancy >42 completed weeks; a baby born after this period

Postnatal period – 'means the period after the end of labour during which the attendance of a midwife upon a woman and baby is required, being not less than 10 days and for such longer period as the midwife considers necessary' (NMC 2004b, *Midwives' Rules and Standards* p. 7)

Postneonatal – period from the end of the neonatal period until the end of the first year

PPH – postpartum haemorrhage – bleeding from the genital tract following the birth of the baby – 500 ml or less if the woman is shocked; primary PPH = during the first 24 hrs; secondary, after this, often 7–14 days

Precipitate labour – sudden onset of labour / rapid delivery of baby

Pre-eclampsia – signs / symptoms possibly leading to eclampsia; fulminating pre-eclampsia = severe condition / imminent eclampsia

Premature rupture of membranes (PROM) – when the membranes rupture spontaneously one hour or more prior to the onset of labour

Prematurity / pre-term – where the pregnancy <37 completed weeks; labour which commences during this time; the resulting baby

Presentation / presenting part – the fetal part lying lowest in the birth canal – felt on abdominal palpation – usually the head (see **abdominal palpation** in Section 2)

Primigravida – a woman pregnant for the first time

Prn – *pro re nata*, as required / indicated, often on prescription

Prolonged labour – lasting longer than expected; previously labour lasting >24 hours in a primigravida but this is now controversial as progress is the main consideration (see **labour** above, and **prolonged labour – first stage** and **prolonged labour – second stage** in Section 2)

PROM (Premature rupture of membranes) – when the membranes rupture spontaneously one hour or more prior to the onset of labour

PU – **passing / passed urine**

Puerperium – a six-week period following the birth of the baby when the pelvic organs return to their original size, shape and site and lactation is established

PV – *per vaginam* – examination, i.e. vaginal examination; or something passed, e.g. blood

RDS – **respiratory distress syndrome**

Reg. – **registrar / senior registrar**, experienced senior doctor

Restitution – where the fetal head rights itself to be aligned with the fetal back during the mechanism of labour

Retained placenta – failed delivery of placenta during third stage of labour – may / may not be separated from uterine wall

Retained products of conception – where products of conception remain in the uterus following miscarriage / birth – may lead to primary / secondary PPH

Retinopathy – condition associated with prematurity – increased vascularisation behind the retina leading to retinal damage and subsequent visual impairment in varying degrees

Retraction ring – occurs in normal labour at the junction of upper and lower segments – upper segment thickens and shortens, lower segment thins and elongates – in obstructed labour the exaggerated retraction ring is palpable above the symphysis pubis – a Bandl's ring

Rhesus factor (Rh) – 'Rhesus-positive' denotes the presence of an antigen on the red blood cells of 85% of the UK population; antibodies built up against this antigen by a Rhesus-negative woman can pass across the placenta and damage Rhesus-positive fetal red blood cells: this is called 'Rhesus incompatibility' (see **anti D immunoglobulin, Kleihauer test, jaundice**)

Rotation – where the fetal head moves round through part of a circle to come under the free space of the pubic arch during the mechanism of labour

Runner, the – operating theatre helper (an auxiliary, health care assistant, student) fetching essential supplies / equipment and dealing with odd jobs during an operation

SANDS – Stillbirth and Neonatal Death Society

Save serum – venous blood is sent to the laboratory in a plain tube, i.e. without an anti-clotting agent. Once the blood is clotted the serum is saved to enable blood to be cross-matched rapidly in an emergency, rather than completing the cross-matching when the blood may not be needed

SB – stillbirth – beware of possible confusion with next abbreviation

SB / SBR – serum bilirubin, i.e. levels of bilirubin in blood – often written on a lab. request form (NB also above use of SB)

SC – subcutaneous – an injection under the skin

SCBU – special care baby unit – less in use today than NNU / NNICU

Schedule drugs – drugs in the five Controlled Drugs Schedules (Misuse of Drugs Regulations 1985), e.g. pethidine, morphine, diamorphine, barbiturates

Schultz method of placental separation – placenta lies in the upper part of the uterus – contraction / retraction reduces placental site, placenta partially separates, the weight causes descent to lower segment, membranes peel off behind it, fetal surface appears at vulva – uterine muscle contraction / retraction mini-mises blood loss (compare with Matthews Duncan separation)

Scriver test (see also **Guthrie test**) – PKU screening test – blood collected on 8–10th day on to filter paper (scc **hccl prick** in Section 2) – overnight electro-phoresis using chemicals allows separation of amino acids according to their molecular weight. Biochemical chromatography (colour) stains separate amino acids, enabling identification of deviations from normal, e.g. phenylketonuria and other inborn errors of metabolism

Scrub – specific hand / lower arm washing technique using antiseptic soap or gel solution, prior to putting on sterile gloves before aseptic / surgical procedures

SDS – surfactant deficiency syndrome

Second-degree tear – perineal trauma involving the vaginal mucosa and skin and both superficial and deep muscles of the perineal body (see **perineal / sur-rounding area trauma** in Section 2)

Sexually transmitted diseases / infections (STD / STIs) – diseases spread by sexual contact (see Section 2 and **infection – maternal, infection – neonatal** and **antenatal screening** in Section 2)

SFD – small for dates, i.e. the baby is SGA / light for dates (see **intrauterine growth retardation** in Section 2)

SGA – small for gestational age, or SFD

SHO – senior house officer, i.e. a junior doctor with some medical experience – many are undertaking obstetric training before beginning work as a GP

Shock – generally temporary state of massive physiological reaction to bodily damage / emotional trauma – characterised by a cold sweat, reduced blood pressure, rapid pulse, and depression of vital processes, e.g. respiration

Shoulder presentation – transverse fetal lie, with shoulder lowermost in the uterus

SIDS – sudden infant death syndrome (see **sudden infant death syndrome** in Section 2)

Sinciput – the brow, i.e. the area from the supra-orbital ridges to the coronal suture

Slow labour – a misleading lay term – the mother is not in established labour, i.e. the active phase of the first stage (see above), but is either in the latent phase or just having regular Braxton Hicks contractions (see above) that are painful

Spalding's sign – gross overlapping of fetal skull bones following death *in utero* (IUD) – manifestation usually takes 48 hours – seen on X-ray (see **intrauterine death** in Section 2)

SPD – symphysis pubis diastasis, i.e. separation of the (bones of the) symphysis pubis joint

SRM or SROM – spontaneous rupture of membranes

Status eclampticus – repeated eclamptic convulsions without resting phase between – life-threatening – may lead to fetal / maternal death (see **eclampsia** in Section 2)

Status epilepticus – serious condition – repeated epileptic convulsions without resting phase between – ? life-threatening to the woman during pregnancy – considered less harmful to the fetus than eclamptic fits (see **epilepsy** in Section 2)

Stillbirth – the complete expulsion of a baby >24 weeks which does not breathe, cry or show any other signs of life (see **intrauterine death** and **Stillbirth and Neonatal Death Society** in Section 2)

Subinvolution – uterus does not involute at the expected rate following delivery – ? result of retained products of conception or blood clots; uterine infection – uterus ? bulky, tender to touch; ? lochia offensive (see **postnatal observations – mother** in Section 2)

Succenturiate lobe – a placenta with an extra cotyledon in the membranes with its own blood supply from the main placenta (see Diagram 5.6)

Supine hypotensive syndrome – compression of the inferior vena cava from the gravid uterus when the woman lies flat on her back – BP falls, woman feels faint, nauseated, is pale / clammy – sitting her up / turning on to left side relieves pressure / allows recovery

Surfactant / surfactant deficiency syndrome (SDS) – a surface activating agent allowing the alveoli to remain expanded when the first breath is taken – absence causes a syndrome (see **respiratory distress syndrome** in Section 2)

Sutures of the fetal skull – incomplete ossification areas, leaving membranous spaces between the skull bones; where more than two suture lines meet = fontanelles

SPD – symphysis pubis diastasis – separation of the (bones of the) symphysis pubis

Syntocinon (*synto*) – synthetic oxytocin – acts quickly on the uterus to produce contractions – used in IVI to induce / augment labour – may also be used intravenously in a single dose in PPH (see **oxytocic drugs, ergometrine, Syntometrine**)

Syntometrine – synthetic oxytocic agent containing 0.5 mg ergometrine and 5 IU (international units) Syntocinon – given IM during the birth of the anterior shoulder (active management, third stage); acts within two minutes, but produces a sustained uterine contraction (see **oxytocic drugs, ergometrine, Syntocinon**)

Tachycardia – increase in the heart rate – adult >100 beats per minute (for example in anaemia or after haemorrhage) – fetal >160 beats per minute (see **fetal distress** in Section 2, and *baseline tachycardia* under **cardiotocography** in Section 2)

Tachypnoea – increase in the respiratory rate – adult >30 per minute – infant >60 per minute; neonatal transient tachypnoea = respiratory rate >60 per minute on a number of occasions without underlying pathology

TBA – traditional birth attendant – (see **Safe Motherhood Initiative** in Section 2)

TCI – 'to come in', i.e. admit to hospital

TDS – three times a day – often on a prescription

TED (thrombo-embolic disorder) stockings – thick elastic stockings (usually white) used to help maintain lower limb support to help prevent DVT

Term / full term – pregnancy that has reached 37 completed weeks gestation: Ellwood (1999) indicates a lack of consensus on the definition, i.e. does it mean 37 + 0 days, or 37 + 7 days, i.e. 38 weeks.

Termination of pregnancy (TOP) – the products of conception are expelled from the uterus by artificial means, i.e. surgically / medically with drugs

Third-degree tear – involves the vaginal mucosa, superficial and deep muscles of the perineal body, and the anal sphincter (see **perineal / surrounding area trauma** in Section 2)

TORCH – acronym for intrauterine infections – toxoplasmosis, others, rubella (a notifiable disease) cytomegalovirus, herpes (see **infection – maternal, infection – neonatal** and **antenatal screening** in Section 2)

Toxaemia – a no-longer accepted term (see **pre-eclampsia**; and **pregnancy-induced hypertension** in Section 2)

Trial of labour – when there is doubt about the ability of the fetal head to pass through the maternal pelvis during labour – effective uterine contractions, descent, flexion and some degree of moulding may enable head progression (see **CPD**)

Trial of scar – labour is allowed to start spontaneously (if possible) in a woman with a caesarean section scar to see if vaginal delivery is achievable – close monitoring of fetal and maternal conditions is essential

Trumpet – refers to the Pinard fetal stethoscope

TSA – **'to see again'**, often written in case notes

TTA, TTH, TTO – **'to take away / home / out'** (of medication)

Tubes – usually refers to a stethoscope

Turner's syndrome – karyotype XO with female characteristics – ? presents with neck webbing, widely angled elbows, protuberant abdomen, lower limb oedema, mental retardation – ? undiagnosed until failure to develop secondary sex characteristics / menstruation in teenage years

U & E – blood test for **urea and electrolytes** to ascertain renal function

US or USS – **ultra sound / ultra sound scan** – echoes of high-frequency sound waves form electronic images of body structures (see **antenatal screening** in Section 2)

UTI – **urinary tract infection**

Valsalva manoeuvre – the woman is asked to take a deep breath in, hold it and push down with all her strength until she cannot push any longer; originally used as a method for expelling pus from the ears; was used as a form of directed pushing until fairly recently

Vasa praevia – where the blood vessels from a succenturiate lobe or velamentous insertion run across the internal os of the cervix when the membranes are intact. If the membranes rupture the blood vessels also rupture, causing fetal haemorrhage

VDRL – **Venereal Disease Reference Laboratory** (see **infection – maternal**, **infection – neonatal** and **antenatal screening** in Section 2)

VE – **vaginal examination**

Velamentous insertion – where the blood vessels from the cord run through the membranes before being inserted into the fetal surface of the placenta (see Diagram 5.5)

Venereal disease (VD) – terminology formerly used for sexually transmitted diseases / infections (STD/ STIs), especially gonorrhoea / syphilis (see **infection – maternal**, **infection – neonatal** and **antenatal screening** in Section 2)

Ventouse – a suction cap made of silicone plastic (silastic). It fits on to the baby's head rather like a skull cap. Once the cap has been positioned, the air is sucked out of it by means of a vacuum. Steady gentle traction during a contraction facilitates the delivery.

Vernix caseosa – white, lard-type substance covering the fetal skin *in utero* to protect against possible damage from being in a watery environment – some may still be present at birth

Version – correction of the fetal presentation; external cephalic version (ECV) – the fetus is pushed head over heels externally (breech to head) before the onset of labour (NICE 2003); internal podalic version – vaginally during labour a transverse lie is converted to breech by pulling a leg down (see **presentation**; and **breech delivery** in Section 2)

Vertex – circular area on skull vault that presents when the head is well flexed; bounded by anterior and posterior fontanelles and parietal eminences on either side (see **abdominal palpation** and **delivery technique** in Section 2)

Viable / viability – capable of independent life = 24 weeks pregnancy in UK

Vital statistics – statistics relating to life, death, disease – UK statistics include the fertility rate, live births, stillbirths, perinatal, neonatal, post-neonatal and infant mortality rates, and maternal mortality / morbidity

VKDB – vitamin K deficiency bleeding (see **haemorrhagic disease** in Section 2)

Zygosity, determining – determining whether twins are identical (monozygous – derived from one single fertilised ovum) or fraternal (dizygous – derived from two different fertilised ova).

Zygote – the cell formed when the nuclear materials of the ovum and sperm unite

Quick Reference Topics

2

This section of the book contains an alphabetical list of a wide variety of quick reference topics from basic midwifery and nursing procedures to obstetric and medical conditions, including emergency situations that may occur during the childbearing continuum. It also contains information on organisations that offer information for parents and professionals on specific conditions, e.g. Down's syndrome, and support services.

Abdominal palpation

Aim:

Assess uterine growth
Determine fetal number, lie, presentation, position, attitude
Assess presenting part engagement
Locate / count fetal heart
Reassure the mother

Preparation:

Inform woman of procedure, gain consent
Ensure her bladder is empty
Expose abdomen from xiphisternum to pubic hair line
Wash hands / stand on the woman's right

Action:

Inspection – size, shape, scars, skin changes, FM
Palpate fundal height – often measured with a tape from symphysis to fundus
Chart fundal height (Gardosi and Francis 1999; NICE 2003)
Fundal palpation – ? head or breech in fundus
Lateral palpation – locate a firm unbroken surface, the back

Pelvic palpation – confirm presentation, assess engagement of presenting part

Auscultation – Pinard's stethoscope – locate fetal heart over fetal back, below maternal umbilicus if head presentation, above if breech presentation; listen to rate, rhythm and volume for 1 minute

Explain findings and encourage mother to feel her baby

Document appropriately

Student activity:
Note the research about assessing fundal height

Active management of labour
Function:

Prevent prolonged labour, maternal / fetal compromise

Reduce instrumental / operative deliveries

Improve woman's personal attention

Assessing / monitoring progress:

Labour onset – accurate labour diagnosis essential

Present contractions – frequency, strength, length, regularity

When / if membranes ruptured

Maternal condition:

    (i)   physical – well-being, pain, vital signs, fluid balance, urinalysis

    (ii) psychological – coping ability, needs / wishes

Fetal condition:

    (i)   FH / CTG (see guideline: NICE 2001a)

    (ii) presenting part position / descent

    (iii) clear / meconium liquor

    (iv) blood pH

VE: progress noted on partograph

If slow, progress of labour augmented / accelerated in uncomplicated cases may become part of a midwife's sphere of practice, depending on local protocols (and see Rule 6 in NMC 2004b)

Administration of drugs
Aim:

Administer medication safely

Keep accurate records

Observe the effects of the medication

Preparation for all methods:

Collect prescription sheet

Check drug administration record to ensure medication not already given

Check each prescribed drug for:
- (i) date prescribed
- (ii) drug name, form, dose, expiry date
- (iii) route of administration
- (iv) specific directions for use
- (v) time(s) due
- (vi) client drug sensitivity
- (vii) doctors signature

Adhere to hospital policy for:
- (i) injection site
- (ii) administration of controlled drugs
- (iii) who can give IV injections

Action:
Oral:
Identify woman / seek consent

Place selected drug in container

Give to woman to take, with a drink prn

Ensure drug swallowed

Record drug administration / response on appropriate chart

IM / SC injection:
Identify woman / seek consent.

Ensure appropriate drug / dosage – check by trained staff

Draw up aseptically / place in receiver

Prepare needle and syringe for injection

Swab skin prn

Insert needle and withdraw plunger to ensure no blood

Administer drug

Observe for effect

Record appropriately

Controlled drug:
Two staff members to check ampoule / tablets

Count stock remaining – record in controlled drugs book

At woman's bedside check ID labels / seek consent

Drug administered as previously

Record drug given in case notes / on prescription sheet

Record in controlled drugs book as given and witnessed

Observe / record effects of medication

Intravenous injections:

Check drug details / dilution / infusion

Check fluid / equipment

Two staff members identify client / seek consent

Ensure appropriate drug / dosage

Draw up aseptically

Administer at prescribed rate, usually through cannula port; sometimes directly IV

Observe / record effects of medication (NB onset likely to be rapid)

Record drug given in case notes / on prescription sheet

Adding to infusion bag:

As for IV injection but:

    (i)   stop infusion

    (ii) add to bag and shake

    (iii) label correctly

    (iv) check infusion rate for administration

    (v) recommence at given rate

Giving via a syringe driver:

As for IV injection but:

    (i)   make volume up with suitable dilution prn

    (ii) prime infusion tube before measuring the barrel length of medication to be infused

    (iii) set rate according to prescribed dose / maker's instructions

    (iv) set / check rate with prescription sheet – start the pump

    (v) check pump, cannula, tubing at least 4-hourly

Student activity:

Ensure you have a copy of Guidelines for the Administration of Medicines (NMC 2002); and Midwives' Rules and Standards (NMC 2004b)

Note your unit policy on drug administration and standing orders

Further reading: Dimond 2002 Chapter 20

Admission in labour

Aim:

Ascertain physical condition

Determine whether labour established

Alleviate fear / anxiety

Facilitate care planning

Offer support prn

Preparation:
Ensure privacy
Read woman's hand-held notes / case record
Ensure maternal / fetal monitoring equipment available

Action:
Follow recorded special instructions
Perform quick assessment – is delivery imminent?
- (1) yes – take straight to delivery room – proceed
- (2) no – explain / complete admission procedure
    - (i)   take history of onset of labour
    - (ii) perform 'top to toe' examination
    - (iii) ask whether bowels open / test urine sample
    - (iv) palpate abdomen
    - (v)   assess contraction frequency, strength, duration, mother's response
    - (vi) VE prn with woman's consent
    - (vii) inform woman and partner of findings
    - (viii) discuss plans for rest of care
    - (ix) keep accurate records
    - (x)   fetal heart monitoring ? routine admission procedure

Student activity:
Note your unit policy for admission, observe records for documenting admission in labour

Adoption
Legislation:
First Adoption Act 1926
Subsequent Acts 1958 and 1968
Children Act 1975 (Part I)
Adoption Act 1976
Children Act 1989
Adoption and Children Act 2002

Welfare Principle:
The child's long- and short-term welfare and wherever possible its feelings

Role of Local Authority:
Has the power to make, and participate in arrangements for the adoption and placing of children who are not in care for adoption.

Supervises children intended for adoption.

Appoints a Guardian *ad litem* as child's advocate, usually an experienced social worker, in a contested adoption or if there are High Court proceedings, and as a court adviser.

Provides counselling service for adoptees wishing to apply for their original birth certificate.

Who Can Adopt?:

Married couples (including same-sex), one of whom must be over 21 and the other over 18 years, unless they are the mother or father of the child.

Must be resident in the UK

Single person over 21 years of age (there must be special grounds for a man to adopt a female child unless he is the partner of the child's mother)

One partner of a pair if the spouse cannot be found or is mentally ill

Children for Adoption:

Must be free for adoption, under 18 and not married.

Parental consent must be given unless:

   (i)   parent dead or missing
   (ii) parent withholding consent unreasonably
   (iii) parent guilty of persistently or seriously ill-treating child
   (iv) child living with adoptive parents for 5 years
   (v)   natural father of child.

Procedure for Adoption:

Parents – both natural and adoptive – *must* understand that it is legal, binding and permanent.

The new Act provides for support services for these parents.

Placement of Child:

With Local Authority Adoption Agency

With Voluntary Adoption Agency (approved)

Direct Placement only if relative of child

Process:

Natural mother contacts Social Services Department or hospital social worker (in pregnancy) regarding adoption – formal consent obtained after baby reaches six weeks.

Doctor certifies mother's general and mental health and provides details of pregnancy, labour and other relevant factors.

Prospective adoptive parents apply to adoption agency.

Adoption Agency investigates prospective parents' suitability; tries to 'match' babies to parents; advises and helps both natural and adoptive parents with legal aspects; respects natural parents' wishes re religious upbringing.

Local Authority must be notified of intention to adopt at least 13 weeks before adoption order can be made, to enable investigations.

Baby for Adoption

Physically examined, any defects noted, adoptive parents informed.

Placed with foster parents or may remain with mother (often in mother and baby unit).

Placed with adoptive parents when **6 weeks** old or possibly on discharged from hospital, but no consent can be given before 6 weeks in case mother changes her mind.

Lives with adoptive parents for **13 weeks**, enabling investigations and home visits and thus ensuring suitability.

The Court (High Court, County Court, Children and Family Court)

Ensures:

    (i)   mother consents to the adoption

    (ii) that adoption is in the best interest of the child

    (iii) that no reward was given to the mother by the adoptive parents.

Appoints the Children and Family Court Advisory and Support Person for the purposes of any relevant application – the officer appointed:

    (i)   acts on behalf of the child and safeguards its interests;

    (ii) prepares a child welfare report;

    (iii) witnesses documents; and

    (iv) performs prescribed functions.

Grants, refuses or postpones for 2 years the Adoption Order, depending on circumstances.

Other Points:

Natural parent needs a court order to remove child living with adoptive parents or foster parents prior to adoption.

If an Adoption Agency is not involved, i.e.: if the child is placed by the High Court or if it is a foster child and consent has been given – child must have lived with adoptive parents for **12 months** as part of the family and must have been visited in the home.

If no parental consent is given, child must have lived with adoptive parents for **5 years**.

If a child is being adopted from another country, then the laws of that country must be followed.

Adoption proceedings will be heard in private.

When 18 the adoptee can apply to the Registrar's Office for information necessary for obtaining his/her original birth certificate.

If a child is placed with an Adoption Agency but is not adopted after one year the natural parents can apply to resume control, but the Court has to be satisfied that the child will be looked after properly. If the parent does not want to resume control – then the LA looks after the child.

The new Act emphasises avoiding delay and the agencies involved in the adoption have to:

(i)   draw up a timetable of events

(ii) provide directions to ensure the timetable is adhered to.

The Act 'tightens up' loopholes so that children do not get lost in the system and are not moved from one carer to another unnecessarily.

Amniocentesis (not a midwife's procedure)

Aim:

Aseptic removal of liquor sample for investigation

Reassure mother / allay fears

Prevent Rhesus incompatibility

Preparation:

Explain procedure to woman / partner

Obtain consent

Ultrasound room ready

Ensure client privacy / safety

Trolley prepared:

(i)   correct pack

(ii)   needles and syringes

(iii) sample bottles

(iv)   local anaesthetic

(v)   dressings / plastic spray

(vi)   cleansing solution

(vii) necessary request forms

Observations of mother / fetus prior to procedure

Action:

Assist doctor with equipment preparation

Reassure mother, act as advocate prn

Assist doctor with procedure prn

Observe mother / fetus following procedure

Keep accurate records

Give IM anti-D immunoglobulin 250 IU if Rhesus negative / status unknown

Escort to ward / couch for rest / observation

Inform woman of signs / symptoms of miscarriage and action to take if present

Student activity:
List indications for performing amniocentesis

Anaemia
A deficiency in the quality or quantity of the red blood cells (rbc) (erythrocytes), and therefore in the oxygen-carrying capacity of the blood. Hb (haemoglobin) of 11.5 g (grams per decilitre, i.e. per 100 ml) during the first trimester or 10.5 g in later pregnancy = anaemia (NICE 2003)

Aetiology:
Iron deficiency – poor diet, malabsorption
Folic acid deficiency
B_{12} deficiency (pernicious anaemia)
Haemoglobinopathies, i.e. abnormal haemoglobin, e.g. sickle cell
Blood loss – acute, i.e. haemorrhage, or chronic, e.g. due to infection
Aplastic anaemia – inability to produce rbc
Blood disorders, e.g. leukaemia

Signs and symptoms:
Possibly asymptomatic, i.e. no obvious symptoms
Tiredness, lethargy
Pallor, i.e. skin and inside of lower eyelid
Breathlessness
Fainting
Tachycardia
Frequent infections

Investigations:
History
Blood film (FBC) – Hb, serum folate, serum ferritin, red cell picture (size, colour, maturity – see **MCH** and **MCV** in Section 1)

Management:
Depends on cause and blood picture
Correct known cause
Iron prn (historically iron was given *routinely* in pregnancy)
Folic acid – all women should have 400 mcg daily before conception and for 1st 12 weeks gestation (NICE 2003)

Possible complications:
Poor general health and resistance to infection
Inability to withstand haemorrhage
Perinatal and maternal mortality / morbidity

Student activity:
Further reading: Ursell 2005

Antenatal screening

All screening is the examination of an asymptomatic population to detect those
likely to develop a condition in whom the disease is already present. There
should be set criteria to determine who should be screened for what. Tests
should be safe, simple, quick and cheap, providing repeatable, valid results.
Antenatal screening is *offered* to all pregnant women, but may lead to anxiety
as well as reassurance.

Routine tests and examinations offered may consist of:

Abdominal examination:

> To determine symphysis–fundal distance to estimate fetal size and growth
> Auscultation to confirm life or at the mother's request (NICE 2003)

Blood pressure measuring:

> Usually at every visit

Weight and height:

> To calculate body mass index (BMI) at booking (NICE 2003)

Urinalysis:

> At every visit for protein and glucose
> MSSU at booking for asymptomatic bacteruria (NICE 2003)

Blood tests:

> ABO and Rhesus group (if Rhesus-negative the partner may be offered
>   screening)
> Rhesus antibodies at booking and 28 weeks
> Haemoglobin at booking and 28 weeks (see **anaemia** in Section 2 above)
> Haemoglobinopathies (see website below)
> Rubella titre (to assess immunity) at booking
> VDRL – for syphilis
> hCG, AFP, uE3, inhibin A (part of Down's syndrome screening – see NICE 2003)
> Hepatitis B (a notifiable disease), hepatitis C
> HIV

Ultrasound scan:

> Ideally 10–13 weeks (NICE 2003) for gestation and nuchal translucency (part of
>   Down's syndrome screening)
> At 18–20 weeks for anomalies

Additional tests offered when necessary:

Amniocentesis (see above)

Biophysical profile (see **fetal distress** below)

Blood sugar (see **diabetes** below)

Chorionic villus sampling (see below)

Haemoglobinopathies (see below)

Vaginal swab for infection, e.g. *Candida*, *Chlamydia*, gonorrhoea

Toxoplasmosis (see **infection – neonatal** below)

Student activity:

Further reading: Bott 2000(a); Emery 2000; http://www.dh.gov.uk http://www. kcl-phs.org.uk/haemscreening/antenatal.htm

Antepartum haemorrhage

Causes:

Lower genital tract:

Infection

Trauma (accident or assault)

Cervical abnormalities, e.g. ectopy (erosion), polyp (small fleshy growth), CIN (see Section 1)

Upper genital tract:

Placental abruption (placenta separating)

Placenta praevia (placenta in the lower uterine segment)

Trauma, e.g. road accident

Uterine rupture

Ruptured vasa praevia (placental vessel in amniotic sac below presenting part)

Predisposing or risk factors:

History of miscarriage, abortion or caesarean section

High parity and older age

Cocaine use and smoking

Hypertensive disorders

Multiple pregnancy

Domestic violence

Management (see Figure 1, p. 31):

Depends on:

    (i)   diagnosis

    (ii) severity of bleeding

    (iii) fetal / maternal conditions.

Not midwife-led care – medical aid in accordance with a midwife's responsibility and sphere of practice (Rule 6 in *Midwives' Rules and Standards*: NMC 2004b)

Antepartum haemorrhage

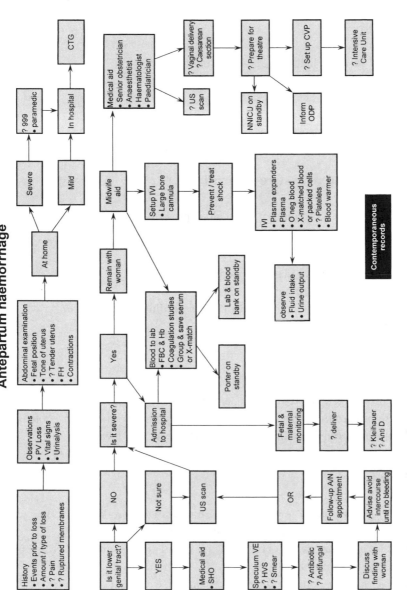

Figure 1 Antepartum haemorrhage

Complications:

Risk of uterine infection

Shock, compromising mother and baby

DIC

Perinatal death

Maternal death

Psychological morbidity, e.g. post-traumatic stress

Student activity:

Note your local policies and procedures for APH

Further reading: Boyle 2002

Arterial blood pressure recording

Aim:

Measure / record / monitor arterial blood pressure

Preparation:

Explain procedure to client / gain consent

Check previous recordings

Check sphygmomanometer (sphyg.) / BP recording device working

Client in suitable position

Action:

Expose arm / palpate antecubital fossa for pulse

Position sphyg. at approximately heart height

Secure cuff around upper arm (ensuring large enough) and inflate – note when
    pulse obliterated and inflate to 20 mmHg above this level

Release valve:

    (i)   systolic BP – first sound

    (ii) diastolic BP – when sound changes, i.e. Korotkoff 4 (K4) or when
        sound disappears, i.e. Korotkoff 5 (K5)

(NB – K4 commonly used in pregnancy for greater accuracy (conflicting views)
– K5 recorded by automated sphyg.)

Electric sphyg. – ensure microphone placed over brachial artery / follow
    instructions

Disconnect equipment

Leave client comfortable

Record findings accurately / inform client

Student activity:

Revise normal BP mechanism control / physiological changes during pregnancy

Further reading: Bennett 1994

Artificial feeds – bottle feeding

Aim:

To ensure formula feeds reconstituted correctly

To reduce the risk of infection due to poor hygiene

To ensure adequate infant nutrition

Preparation:

Prepare clean working surface

Explain procedure to mother

Ensure equipment sterilised

Boil water – allow to cool to a maximum of hand-hot

Wash hands

Action:

Remove bottles / teats from sterilizer, ensuring no contamination

Read instructions on side of formula packet – determine quantity of feed required

Put correct amount of *cooled* boiled water into bottle

Using scoop provided, fill with powder and level off with knife

Put scoop of powder into bottle, repeat prn

Put cap and teat on, shake vigorously

Allow to cool, test temperature on inside of wrist before giving

If several bottles being made up, put teats inside bottle

Once at room temperature, store in 'fridge' until required

Ensure mother understands baby should be held during feed and not 'propped up' in a pushchair / cot

Student activity:

Familiarise yourself with reports on infant feeding and Baby Friendly Initiative (see also **Breast Feeding Initiative (BFI)** below)

Artificial rupture of membranes (ARM) (forewater amniotomy) (also see **augmentation /acceleration of labour** in Section 1 and **induction of labour – alternative and 'natural'** and **induction of labour – medical** in Section 2 below)

Aim:

Rupture forewaters in order to accelerate labour

To exclude abnormalities, e.g. meconium liquor

Preparation:

Ensure privacy / maintain dignity

Explain procedure / seek consent (NMC 2004a)

Trolley prepared

Dressing pack

Sterile cleansing solution

Device for rupturing membranes (Amnihook / amnicot)

Sterile pads

Pinard's stethoscope / sonicaid

Abdominal palpation

Comfortable position

Action:

Woman's bladder should be empty, vulva exposed

Aseptic technique

Swab vulva

Vaginal examination – confirm:

    (i)   dilatation of cervix

    (ii) presenting part

    (iii) no cord present

    (iv) forewaters intact

With two fingers of right hand in vagina:

    (i)   guide device to forewaters avoiding vaginal trauma

    (ii)   wait for contraction and bulging forewaters (if possible)

    (iii) rupture membranes

    (iv) remove device, avoiding trauma

    (v)   fetal scalp electrode (FSE) applied prn

    (vi) check liquor draining / clear

    (vii) exclude cord prolapse

    (viii) remove fingers / place clean pad over vulva

Listen to fetal heart

Advise mother of findings and make comfortable

Record procedure accurately, including indications for ARM

Aseptic technique

Aim:

Reduce contamination risk during procedures

Preparation:

Inform client of procedure / gain consent (NMC 2004a)

Clean dressing trolley – from top downwards

Sterile solution / other necessary equipment on lower shelf

Place sterile pack on top of trolley – check expiry date

Open carefully, secure outer bag to trolley for disposal of swabs

Ensure privacy / maintain client dignity

Action:

Wash hands

Open inner pack carefully / prepare equipment prn

Maintain clean field / area of appropriate body part

Wash hands again or use surgical rub

Use sterile gloves / forceps for procedure

Dispose of soiled swabs / forceps safely

Document actions / observations

Ensure client comfortable following procedure

Augmentation / acceleration of labour (also see induction of labour – alternative and 'natural' and induction of labour – medical below)

Medically enhancing spontaneous labour when progress slow / failed

ARM (see above) and IV cannulation may be part of the midwife's sphere of practice (see Rule 6: NMC 2004a, *Midwives' Rules and Standards*)

First identify cause: (see **prolonged labour** – first stage below)

Contraindications	*Cautious use*
major CPD	minor CPD
malpresentation	multigravidas
multiple pregnancy	uterine scar
severe APH	IUGR / compromised fetus
	unstable lie

Methods:

ARM (forewater amniotomy) – once performed delivery is committed

Indications:	*Contraindications*
with woman's informed consent	if women objects
labour established	spurious labour – i.e., not established
cervix 4 cm or more dilated	cervix <4 cm dilated
slow progress	high presenting part
inadequate contractions	complications
for liquor examination	
application of FSE	

Advantages of ARM
? shortens labour (no consensus in
research)
liquor observation
FSE application
? closer application of cervix to head
may increase dilatation and
stimulate prostaglandin release

Disadvantages of ARM
stress and anxiety during procedure
cervical / vaginal wall trauma
fetal hypoxia from cord compression /
prolapse
fetal bradycardia due to fall in
placental perfusion / head
compression
maternal shock if sudden large
drainage
discomfort from draining liquor
caput / cephalhaematoma formation
excess moulding
increased frequency / strength of
contractions
increased pain / less able to cope /
more analgesia
increased risk of intrauterine infection
maternal / neonatal infection
woman may feel a lack of control /
decreased satisfaction

Possible advantages of intact membranes
labour not committed
even pressure on fetus during contractions
less risk of infection
? pain more tolerable

Syntocinon added to IVI
With woman's informed consent (NMC 2004a)
Administered via an infusion pump for dose accuracy
Before ARM or following ARM
Initial slow rate gradually increases
stimulates uterine contractions to accelerate labour

Advantages
shortens labour
gives some control over labour
readily stopped if complications
increases chances of
spontaneous vaginal
delivery

Disadvantages
increased frequency / strength of
contractions
increased pain / less able to cope / more
analgesia
continuous electronic fetal monitoring often
applied
lessens mobility / alternative positions

over-stimulation / tonic contractions

fluid overload (oxytocin has anti-diuretic properties)

? increases neonatal jaundice

Management:

Close monitoring of fetal / maternal well-being

? Continuous electronic fetal monitoring (see **CTG** in Section 1) (NICE 2001a, 2001b)

Maternal vital signs

Fluid balance

Urinalysis for ketones

IVI gradually increased – contractions maximum 1:3 to 4 – ?decreased as progressing

Ensure uterus relaxes between contractions

Close monitoring of progress – contractions; abdominal examination; VE

Usual care in labour

? Oral ranitidine (see **Mendelson's syndrome** below)

? Only clear fluids orally

Information / support for woman / partner

Continue Syntocinon infusion for 1 hour after delivery (<PPH)

Student activity:

Note your local policy and procedures

Familiarise yourself with labour records

Revise physiology of labour

Further reading: Arulkumaran and Symonds 1999

Birth asphyxia (see **fetal distress** in Section 2 and **Apgar score** in Section 1)

Failure to establish spontaneous breathing – with / without heartbeat. The Apgar score is commonly utilised to determine severity of neonatal compromise (see Figure 4, p. 80).

Aetiology:

Obstructed airway – liquor; mucus; blood; meconium

Respiratory depression, e.g. due to pethidine, morphine, or GA

Cerebral haemorrhage

Congenital abnormalities, e.g. heart, lungs

Prematurity – lack of surfactant in lungs (RDS); immature respiratory centre / system

Severe intrauterine infection

Pneumothorax (air in chest) or reflex apnoea due to mismanaged initial resuscitation

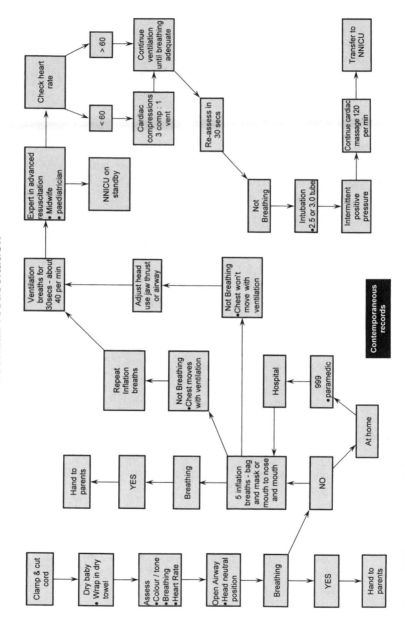

Figure 2 Neonatal resuscitation

Management:
> Neonatal resuscitation see Figure 2, p. 38.

Bladder care in labour

Aim:
> Prevent bladder damage during labour
> Prevent full bladder delaying progress
> Detect abnormalities in urine, e.g. ketones

Preparation:
> Ensure privacy / maintain dignity
> Collect equipment prn – e.g. bed pans, urinalysis sticks
> Inform woman about emptying bladder at regular intervals

Action:
> Early labour encourage mobilisation and fluids prn
> Empty bladder 2–4 hourly, perform and record urinalysis
> If not mobile – offer bedpans at regular intervals 2–4 hourly
> If full bladder palpated / unable to empty – catheterise
> Prior to caesarean section – ? insert an indwelling catheter
> Prior to instrumental delivery – ? catheterisation (non-retaining)

Student activity:
Describe why a full bladder may cause problems in labour; how may damage to
the bladder be minimised?

Blood glucose monitoring (neonatal) – see heel prick in Section 2

Blood pressure measuring – see arterial blood pressure recording
in Section 2

Bowel care in labour

Aim:
> Prevent full rectum delaying labour progress
> Maintain dignity during the second stage of labour

Preparation:
> During admission ask if her bowels opened prior to labour onset
> Explain importance of empty bowel in labour
> Seek consent if action necessary

Action:

Collect receiver for equipment:

(i)   suppository / enemette

(ii) gloves, lubricating gel / warm water, gauze swabs

(iii) bedpan and cover (unless toilet very close)

(iv) bedding protection

Ensure privacy

Woman in left lateral position, knees bent, buttocks exposed

Protect bedding

Suppository:

Lubricate (lubricant on gauze)

Locate anus, insert suppository 4.5 cm into the rectum using gloved index finger

Instruct woman to hold suppository for as long as possible

Enemette:

Read instructions – snip off top with clean scissors

Lubricate end (lubricant on gauze); insert into anus

Squeeze the contents into the rectum

Cover the woman and leave as comfortable as possible

Ensure call bell within easy reach

Record administration, monitor effectiveness / results

NB – If labour well established, perform VE prior to procedure

Breast expression of milk

NB not part of normal lactation management – may be performed if:

(i)   baby separated from the mother in SCBU

(ii) baby is unable to 'fix' correctly at the breast

(iii) mother wishes to learn technique prior to return to work while maintaining breastfeeding

(iv) temporary medical indication, e.g. drug therapy

(v)   temporary relief of milk engorgement (see **breastfeeding** below)

Aim:

Remove milk from the breast as comfortably as possible.

Prevent breast engorgement.

Preparation:

Explain procedure to mother / seek consent (NMC 2004a)

Equipment sterilised – electric / hand pump, cups, tubing, container for milk

Wash nipples prn

Maintain privacy

Action:

Mechanical / electric pump:

Place cup over nipple and areola.

Apply suction – check not too uncomfortable

Check the milk is being ejected into the correct place

When breast fully expressed, stop suction, remove cup carefully, repeat on other breast

Manual expression:

Carried out by midwife / mother if no pump available / woman prefers

Seat woman comfortably – bed table / similar underneath breast

Place sterile receiver beneath breast to catch milk

Working from the periphery, both hands either side of the breast, massage with firm strokes towards the nipple

Compress the areola and eject the milk into the receiver

As one breast releases milk, the other may also leak – receiver / breast pad in place

If the milk is being saved:

  (i) place in a sterile bottle

  (ii) cover

  (iii) label

  (iv) refrigerate / freeze

Student activity:

Note your local policies

Further reading: Bick 1999; Department of Health 1996a; Jones 1995; Lang 1994; Nikodem *et al.* 1993; Tiran and Mack 1995; Webb 1992; West and Topping 2000

Breastfeeding

Aids to successful breastfeeding:

Atmosphere:

Relaxed, unhurried, private, no interruptions

Rest, family and professional support

Frequency:

Ideally within 1 hour delivery

Babies vary – 1–8 hours, average 3–4 hours

Time suckling according to milk amount / flow, baby's appetite

Foremilk (early flow) higher water and lower fat than more satisfying hindmilk

Position – mother:

Comfortable, relaxed (essential)

Upright, supported by pillows (aids relaxation)

Support arm holding baby (pillows on lap, on raised thigh – foot stool useful)

Lateral position if there are perineal or abdominal wounds

Position – baby:

Head on upper arm, body across mother's chest or vertically, with baby's nearest arm tucked round mother's chest under her arm OR 'back to front', i.e. body under arm, buttocks on a pillow with arm across chest, baby's head positioned for clear nostrils

Breast:

? Supported and/or lifted from below

Point nipple at roof of baby's mouth – if no rooting reflex, stroke the baby's lips with nipple, or cheek with finger

Nipple and areola, especially underside, need to be grasped and drawn into baby's mouth

? Support heavy breast with cupped hand (prevents loss of fixing)

If incorrectly fixed may cause pain – release vacuum using little finger in corner of mouth and press baby's jaw

If correct fixing generally no discomfort to mother and small cheek muscle movement seen in front of baby's ear

Ensure correct fixing after baby pauses

Diet:

No set restrictions

Anecdotal evidence suggests that certain foods may give baby wind / colic/ loose stools:

    (i)   very spicy foods

    (ii) highly acid foods, e.g. pickles and citric fruit / juices

    (iii) large quantities of chocolate

    (iv) some fruit and vegetables

Effects seem to appear 6–48 hours after maternal consumption.

Alcohol levels in milk = maternal plasma levels – therefore minimal intake advised

Tobacco chemicals and metabolites present in milk if mother actively / passively smokes.

Drugs:

The mother should inform her doctor or pharmacist before taking any medication.

This following list is not exhaustive, but includes drugs that are in common use.

Contraindicated	*Caution*
Aspirin	antidepressants (high doses)
Oestrogen, e.g. combined oral contraceptive	antihistamines
tetracycline	co-trimoxazole (Septrin) antibiotics
vitamins A and D in high doses	antimalarials
anti-cancer drugs	corticosteroids (high doses)
	phenobarbitone

Safe

antacids and bulk laxatives
antibiotics – cephalosporins (Ceporex) erythromycin, nystatin, penicillins
anticoagulants – heparin, warfarin
ergometrine
insulin
metronidazole (Flagyl) (normal doses)
paracetamol
progesterone-only contraceptives
vitamins B and C, folic acid
vitamins A and D (normal doses)

Complications:

Information, encouragement and practical tips aid the overcoming of difficulties / continuation of breastfeeding

Nipples:	*Solutions*:
non-protractile (flat) or inverted – likely to make fixing difficult	manual or electronic breast pump may draw nipple out sufficiently to enable baby to fix
	soft nipple shield (sterilised); but this may reduce stimulation / milk transfer
	express milk using pump (see above) and cup / spoon feed
sore / cracked, commonly owing to incorrect fixing (NB if nipple bleeding baby may vomit blood	rest nipple – express milk and cup feed change in mother's/baby's position – correct fixing soft nipple shield as above

(mother's) following a feed);
caution: thrush (*Candida*) may
develop in nipple, increasing
pain

anecdotal evidence suggests nipple
cream may be soothing; antifungal
creams if *Candida* suspected;
breastfeeding on one breast only

Engorgement:

(a) temporary vascular
engorgement due to increased
blood supply in days 2–4 –
breasts feel uniformly tender
/ painful, enlarged and possibly
hot; ? slight, transient pyrexia

Solutions:
warm bathing in bath / shower;
hot and then cold compresses;
well-supporting bra;
mild analgesic, e.g. paracetamol;
dark green cabbage leaves in bra lessen
swelling (Nikodem *et al.* 1993; Tiran
and Mack 1995)

(b) milk engorgement due to
blockage / failure of emptying –
commonly due to incorrect
positioning, occasionally to
greater supply than demand –
breasts may be generally /
locally hard, tender / painful,
hot / inflamed; blocked ampulla
will feel like hard, pea-sized
swellings, causing tenderness
behind areola (NB be aware of
mastitis – pyrexia; generally
unwell; local pain; heat and
inflammation – medical aid
and antibiotics)

correct fixing and / or change of baby's
position hand-express some milk to
soften breast, enabling easier fixing
warm bathing in bath / shower
gentle massage with flat of hand all
round breast to nipple before /
between feeding – hand-express, but
avoid over-stimulation (see below)
homeopathic remedies (Webb 1992)
continue feeding if no pus

Insufficient milk

Considered if baby continually unable to settle and wanting feeding (not just now
and again) and has a low urine output (disposable nappies may make observation of output difficult). May be due to inadequate breast development during
pregnancy due to poor pituitary or placental hormone levels.

Cause	Solutions
poor lactation	correct fixing and frequent feeding aids stimulation
ineffective draught (let down) reflex due to inefficient neurohormonal regulation from:	plenty of rest and relaxation aided by supportive family
(i) inadequate nipple stimulation due to poor fixing	aromatherapy may be useful nutritious diet and adequate fluids

(ii) psychological factors inhibiting hormonal release, e.g. tiredness, stress and anxiety family pressure not to breastfeed

avoid complementary/supplementary feeds if possible – water or formula only if really necessary using cup or spoon feeding
reflexology (Tiran and Mack 1995)
homeopathic remedies (Webb 1992)

Breast Feeding Initiative (BFI)

Set up in 1991 by WHO and UNICEF (United Nations Children's Fund) promoting breastfeeding internationally. The initiative recommends Ten Steps to Successful Breastfeeding, while discouraging adverse practices. The Baby Friendly Hospital Initiative implements this policy, with 'Baby Friendly Hospital' status awarded if external assessors agree that the ten steps have been successfully completed.

Breech

Types:

Complete (flexed) – fetal knees and hips flexed, feet close to buttocks
Extended (frank) – knees extended, feet by head
Footling – one / both feet below buttocks (more common pre-term)
Knee presentation – one / both knees below buttocks (uncommon)

Positions:

Left / right sacro-anterior (LSA / RSA)
Left / right sacro-posterior (LSP / RSP)

Aetiology:

Common in early pregnancy, therefore pre-term birth
Restriction of space and/or ability to turn due to:

(i)   firm abdominal and uterine muscles, e.g. primigravida
(ii) uterine anomalies, e.g. fibroids; bicornuate
(iii) oligohydramnios
(iv) contracted pelvis
(v)   multiple pregnancy
(vi) extended breech

Excess space in uterus:

(i)   lax abdominal and uterine muscles, e.g. grand(e) multiparity
(ii) polyhydramnios

Fetal causes:

(i)   hydrocephalus
(ii) IUD
(iii) IUGR and decreased fetal activity
(iv) short umbilical cord

Diagnosis:

History:

Previous breech

Maternal discomfort under ribs

Fetal movements low in uterus

Abdominal palpation:

Not always easy, especially if breech deeply engaged / legs extended

Presenting part feels less round, bony and ballottable

Fundal part (head) hard, round and ballottable

FH found above umbilicus (except when deeply engaged)

Ultrasound scan

X-ray

Vaginal examination in labour:

presenting part may be high / soft

Anal fissure, anus, sacrum may be felt (meconium on examining finger)

Soft genitalia felt (difficult)

Feet may be felt

Management – in pregnancy:

After 32–34 weeks, obstetric referral

Promotion of spontaneous version (see Further reading):

  (i)   Alexander technique

  (ii) acupuncture

  (iii) knees–chest position

36 weeks to term – ? external cephalic version (ECV) (NICE 2003)

Persistent breech – decision on mode of delivery assisted by:

  (i)   clinical judgement

  (ii) maternal wishes

  (iii) history

  (iv) fetal size, gestation, condition (US scan)

  (v)   size, shape of pelvis (pelvimetry)

Mode of delivery: (see **Term Breech Trial** below)

Elective caesarean section common

Spontaneous or assisted vaginal delivery – in urgent cases (see below) by a
midwife (see *EU Second Midwifery Directive 80/155/EEC* in NMC 2004b)

Management of labour:

Generally in hospital – senior obstetric supervision

If at home (mother's informed choice) inform supervisor of midwives.

Anaesthetist / paediatrician on standby

? Induction of labour

Continuous electronic monitoring usual.

Normal labour care

Clear fluids orally (anaesthetic risk)

? Mobile (aids descent of breech) or bed rest (debatable)

Usual analgesia (epidural prevents premature pushing and entrapment of fetal head in incompletely dilated cervix)

Allow spontaneous rupture of membranes (VE to exclude cord prolapse)

Complications:

Pre-labour rupture of membranes

Cord prolapse

Genital tract bruising / oedema

Placental separation in second stage

Fetal hypoxia due to:
- (i)   cord compression
- (ii) placental separation
- (iii) inhalation of liquor, blood, mucus

Entrapment of head in incompletely dilated cervix

Undiagnosed CPD

Intracranial haemorrhage due to:
- (i)   anoxia
- (ii) tentorial tear

Trauma from faulty handling, e.g.
- (i)   fractures
- (ii) dislocations
- (iii) muscle / nerve damage
- (iv) ruptured abdominal organs

Perinatal mortality

Breech delivery:

Part of a midwife's role in an emergency (NMC 2004b): the midwife must remember the following points:
- (i)   medical aid – obstetrician / paediatrician
- (ii) malpresentation means high risk of mortality / morbidity
- (iii) ensure cervix fully dilated
- (iv) keep hands off the breech as much as possible
- (v)   ensure slow, controlled delivery of head

Aim:

> Safe delivery of baby and placenta
> Minimise traumatic delivery for mother / baby

Preparation:

> Explain breech delivery to mother
> Seek co-operation
> Ensure maternal bladder / rectum empty

Action:

> Encourage mother to push
> Allow spontaneous delivery of buttocks
> Release legs as necessary
> When umbilicus delivered, pull down cord loop, avoiding traction
> Allow weight of body to cause further descent
> Feel for / help deliver elbows / arms
> Wait for shoulders to rotate into antero-posterior diameter (use Løvset's manoeuvre if this fails to occur – see below)
> Grasp baby by iliac crests; tilt towards the maternal sacrum, releasing anterior shoulder
> Lift buttocks towards maternal abdomen, enabling posterior shoulder to deliver
> Allow the body to hang, enabling the head to flex; continue with Burns–Marshall manoeuvre (if the head remains deflexed, continue with Mauriceau–Smellie–Veit manoeuvre, i.e. jaw flexion and shoulder traction encourages head flexion)

Burns–Marshall manoeuvre

> When the hairline appears
> With a finger between the ankles keep the legs extended
> Take legs through 180° arc towards mother until mouth and nose appear at vulva
> Right hand guards perineum until head can be slowly delivered; ? clear airways

Mauriceau–Smellie–Veit manoeuvre

> Straddle baby over the right arm, middle finger in baby's mouth
> Other fingers either side over the cheeks
> Left hand over baby's neck, middle finger splinting neck
> Other fingers over each shoulder
> Apply traction with right hand; push with left hand

Head is slowly flexed

When face free, deliver vault slowly

Løvset's manoeuvre

Grasp baby by iliac crests

Rotate body through half a circle with the back upwards

Posterior shoulder to symphysis – shoulder and arm are freed

Rotate body in reverse direction to release second shoulder and arm

Following delivery of the head:

Give syntometrine (unless contraindicated)

Cut cord, wrap baby, show to mother / take to Resuscitaire

Deliver placenta / membranes (see **delivery technique** (management of third stage of labour) below)

Observe for perineal trauma

Carry out maternal / neonatal observations

Contemporaneous records

Student activity:

Discover if ECV is performed in your unit and observe procedure

Note local policies re management of labour

Review birth register – how many breech deliveries conducted by midwives?

Practice procedure using fetal doll and obstetric model / pelvis

Further reading: Albrechtsen *et al.* 1997 and Lindqvist *et al.* 1997 (mode of delivery); Annapoora *et al.* 1997 (ECV); Machover 1995 (spontaneous version); Coates 2003; Hannah *et al.* 2000; NICE 2003 (ECV)

Brow presentation (see also **OP position** in Section 1)

Head presenting midway between flexion and extension

Diagnosis:
Abdominal examination:

High presenting part

Diameter of head may feel large

? Groove felt between head and back

Vaginal examination:

High presenting part possibly not felt

Orbital ridges and anterior fontanelles felt

USS

Management:

Emergency caesarean section – if 13 cm mentovertical diameter enters pelvic brim head arrests in cavity, i.e. there is obstructed labour

Vaginal delivery if full head extension / flexion leads to face or vertex presentation

Caesarean section

Elective caesarean section:

When vaginal delivery is not considered to be in the mother's / baby's best interests, e.g. in cases of cephalo-pelvic disproportion, placenta praevia, severe pre-eclampsia / PIH

Emergency caesarean section:

When adverse conditions / emergency (e.g. cord prolapse) arise in labour – if anticipated, woman should be forewarned of possibility

Aim – pre-operative care:

Facilitate caesarean section delivery

Support the woman / partner prn

Ensure informed consent gained in writing (NMC 2004a)

Assist obstetrician / paediatrician

Ensure good recovery of mother / baby

Preparation – elective:

Locate / identify woman correctly – presence of ID band

Check woman's understanding of procedures / operation – consent form signed with doctor

Blood to lab. for save serum / X-match prn and clotting screening prn, e.g. in PIH / pre-eclampsia? Arrange a visit to NNU

Ensure appropriate charts labelled

Prescription sheet written up for premedication / post-operative analgesia

Procedures:

(i) woman fasted minimum of 6 hours prior to surgery

(ii) antacids, skin preparation, bowel care given as policy

(iii) bath / shower prior to surgery

(iv) IV infusion sited prn

Complete pre-op. checklist, e.g.:

(1) note:

(i) blood results, i.e. ABO and Rh. Grouping, FBC and Hb, clotting screening prn

    (ii)   observations e.g. urinalysis, TPR and BP, FH / CTG

    (iii) allergies, e.g. drugs, metals, Elastoplast

    (iv) choice of baby names

    (v)   dental bridges / caps present

    (vi) consent form signed

(2) remove:

    (i)   dentures

    (ii)   contact lens(es)

    (iii) jewellery – wedding ring may remain – cover with adhesive tape

    (iv) make-up / nail polish

    (v)   hearing aid – ? removed after woman anaesthetised, to remain with her

Action:

Ask woman to empty bladder – catheter inserted under GA

Give theatre gown / cap to put on

Help with TED stockings prn (see Section 1)

Follow special instructions

Give premedication as prescribed – ensure safety whilst woman under its influence

Inform woman of estimated time of surgery

Assist partner to prepare for theatre if attending delivery

Escort to theatre

Hand over case records / other relevant documentation to theatre staff

Pre-op. check list may be repeated

Preparation / action – emergency:

Pre-op. care minimal

Consent forms signed

IV infusion sited

Observations performed

Support woman / partner – emergency caesarean section possibly a frightening experience

Note choice of baby names

Bladder emptied – catheter commonly inserted under GA

NNU on standby

Immediate post-operative care:

Recovery from anaesthesia in operating theatre recovery area

Close observation of:

    (i)   airway / breathing – ? pulse oximetry for oxygen levels

    (ii) pulse and BP – ? continuous electronic monitoring

(iii) blood loss *per vaginam*

(iv) pain levels

(v) levels of consciousness

If spinal / epidural anaesthesia mother usually alert, but still requires careful observation

Mother / baby contact as soon as possible

Information / support partner

Transferred to the ward when condition stable

Continued post-operative care:

(NB – this is major abdominal surgery + uterine involution / reversal of pregnancy changes)

Ensure satisfactory post-operative recovery

Give adequate analgesia

Encourage development of mother–baby relationship

Assist mother to achieve self-care / return to normal function

Help with baby care / adjustment to motherhood

Preparation:

Bed prepared to receive post-operative client

Observation charts / equipment (for IV infusion, urinary drainage bag / stands) prn

Cot prepared

Nurse-call system accessible

Ensure privacy

Action:

Receive woman / baby to ward

Check identification labels

Note special instructions

Commence post-operative observations:

(i) ? hourly pulse, blood pressure and respirations initially – then four-hourly

(ii) palpate uterine fundus – ensure well contracted

(iii) wound for leakage

(iv) loss *per vaginam*

(v) urinary output / remove catheter as instructed

Encourage leg movement / breathing exercises

Ensure adequate analgesia – ? patient-controlled (PCA) / opiates IM 4–6-hourly

Encourage ambulation as early as condition allows – adequate rest needed

Assist with feeding baby
Encourage contact with baby to promote a good relationship
Offer support / advice prn
If emergency section – ? de-briefing needed
Normal postnatal care as mother recovers
Accurate records

Cardiotocography (CTG)

Simultaneous electronic monitoring of fetal heart and uterine contractions – recorded on special paper rotating at 1 cm per minute

Types:

External:

Doppler ultrasound transducer on mother's abdomen (over most audible FH); pressure-sensitive transducer on maternal abdomen over uterine fundus

Internal:

Fetal scalp electrode (FSE) on presenting part (breech / head) records ECG
Intrauterine catheter (rarely used) records contractions

Indications for use:

All 'high risk' cases during pregnancy (periodic) and labour (continuous) (see NICE 2001(a) guidelines)
Routine on admission in labour (for 20–30 min) (controversial)
Routine during labour (periodic / continuous) (controversial)

Aims:

Detection of fetal compromise, enabling prompt delivery and preventing fetal trauma – evidence / research about efficiency / benefits in labour inconclusive – much discussion about professionals' interpretative ability; also is fetal distress in labour an indication of compromise *prior* to labour?

FH patterns:

Normal baseline rate = 110–160 beats per minute (bpm)

Baseline variability = variation in rate over 10–20 seconds, i.e. 5–15 bpm

Accelerations = FH rate rises for 15 seconds in response to activity / stimulation, e.g. contractions, noise, application of FSE – 2 accelerations in 20 minutes = reactive trace and positive sign of fetal well-being

Baseline bradycardia = a persistent low rate >100 and <110 bpm, uncomplicated if without other indications – ensure recording not of maternal origin – <100 bpm + other CTG / clinical indications = compromised fetus caused by:

  (i)   regional analgesia (epidural), especially if maternal hypotension
  (ii)   congenital heart defects
  (iii) acute hypoxia during contraction, ? transient chemoreceptor-mediated bradycardia (or prolonged deceleration)
  (iv)   excessive uterine activity
  (v)   hypovolaemia following prolonged labour (usually mild)
  (vi)   maternal hypotension due to:
         (a) aortocaval compression (supine hypotension)
         (b) epidural
         (c) shock

Baseline tachycardia = persistently >160 bpm – uncomplicated unless other CTG or clinical indications
Caused by:

  (i)   fetal activity / stimulation, e.g. pain
  (ii)   prematurity < 32–34 weeks
  (iii) drugs to stop pre-term labour
  (iv)   fetal anaemia, especially Rh isoimmunisation
  (v)   fetal bleeding, e.g. vessel puncture in amniocentesis, trauma in vasa praevia
  (vi)   following prolonged deceleration (in response to catecholamine production)
  (vii) maternal pyrexia – infection; prolonged labour; epidural
  (viii) maternal distress
  (ix)   maternal hyperthyroidism

Reduced variability (smooth trace) – 10 min reduction insignificant – observe for 40–50 min period; but >180 min. = fetal acidosis, caused by:

  (i)   prematurity
  (ii)   fetal sleep
  (iii) maternal narcotic, sedative, antihypertensive, general anaesthetic
  (iv)   fetal hypoxia, e.g. in IUGR
  (v)   placental insufficiency, e.g. due to multiple infarcts
  (vi)   oxytocin – increased contractions may lower utero-placental perfusion
  (vii) fetal malformation, e.g. CNS and heart
  (vii) viral infection

However, cases of low variability have resulted in normal outcome.

High variability = >25 bpm caused by:
- (i)   external stimulation
- (ii) cord compression and acute hypoxia

Early decelerations = a decrease in fetal heart rate before or at the beginning of a contraction, rapid return to normal after contraction caused by rapid progression in labour / descent of head due to:
- (i)   fetal head compression
- (ii) raised intracranial pressure and vagal nerve response

Late decelerations = decreased rate after onset of contraction with lowest point after peak of contraction = fetal compromise caused by:
- (i)   uteroplacental insufficiency
- (ii) fetal hypoxia

Variable decelerations = variable in timing, frequency and depth – usually short duration may / may not indicate acute hypoxia (depending on length and depth) caused by:
- (i)   cord compression
- (ii) pressure over orbital ridges, e.g. in breech, posterior position, CPD

Physiology of variable decelerations in healthy fetus:
As cord compresses, vein compresses first; BP falls; this stimulates baroreceptors in autonomic nervous system, so FH goes up
Cord arteries then compress; increased pressure stimulates baroreceptors; then FH falls
As artery pressure comes off, FH rises above normal
As all pressure comes off, FH returns to normal

Sinusoidal pattern = a regular undulating waveform above and below normal baseline rate – 2–5 cycles per minute; absent short-term variability and reactivity – may be typical or atypical, caused by:
- (i)   not fully understood
- (ii)   ? absent neural control of heart
- (iii) ? brain stem hypoxia
- (iv)   fetal anaemia – Rh isoimmunisation; fetal bleeding; feto-maternal haemorrhage
- (v)   severe hypoxia
- (vi)   thumb sucking (seen on scan); pattern only short-term

Discussion:

Clinical situation *must* be considered along with CTG, e.g.

- (i) history – general and obstetric
- (ii) maternal condition – general, antenatal, intrapartum
- (iii) gestation (< 28 weeks FH variations are unreliable – immature fetal autonomic nervous system)
- (iv) uterine contractions, labour stage and progress
- (v) clear / meconium liquor
- (vi) fetal blood sample

Student activity:

Revise the mechanism of heart-rate control.

Note your local policy on antenatal and intrapartum CTG use.

Familiarise yourself with your unit equipment.

Further reading: Herbst and Ingemarsson 1994; Mead 1996; Mitchell 1995; Nelson *et al.* 1996; NICE 2001(a); Symons 1998; Walsh 1998

Carpal tunnel syndrome

Signs and symptoms:

'Pins and needles' / numbness in the fingers.

Aetiology:

Local oedema compressing median nerve in carpal tunnel at the wrist

Usually resolves postnatally as oedema subsides

Management:

If severe, physiotherapist referral

Exercises / supporting splint

Catheterisation

Aim:

Empty the bladder with minimum discomfort

Leave the catheter *in situ* prn

Preparation:

Clean area to work on

Catheterisation pack

Appropriate-sized catheter – narrow lumen if in labour

Sterile gloves

Cleansing solution

Ampoule of sterile water and syringe if in-dwelling catheter

Local anaesthetic gel may be used
Urinary drainage bag, specimen bottle prn
Ensure privacy, seek consent, explain procedure

Action:

Aseptic technique (see above) – use sterile gloves
Protect the bed, open pack, apply gloves
Swab vulva
Local anaesthetic gel may be applied to end of catheter
Separate labia, locate urethra (not always easy in labour; aim 2.5 cm below clitoris)
Insert catheter gently into urethra – ? as much as 10 cm in labour (fetal head may interfere with catheter passage)
Collect urine into receiver and measure – ? collect specimen for laboratory
Remove catheter or fill balloon with sterile water and connect to closed drainage system if catheter indwelling
Make woman comfortable
Accurate records

Cephalo-pelvic disproportion (CPD)

Aetiology:

Large fetus, e.g. genetic origin / maternal diabetes
Small pelvis – ? woman small stature
Abnormal pelvis:
      (i)   non-gynaecoid shape
      (ii) disease, e.g. rickets / osteomalacia
      (iii) fracture, e.g. road accident
      (iv) spinal deformity
Malposition, e.g. occipito-posterior

Consider diagnosis – during pregnancy if:

Non-engaged fetal head in primigravida at 38 weeks / multigravida at term
Abnormal presentation, e.g. breech
Previous prolonged / difficult labour / delivery

Consider diagnosis – during labour if:

Head slow to progress in labour, i.e.
      (i)   slow / halted cervical dilatation
      (ii) head advancement slow in second stage – ? deep transverse arrest (DTA) – (see **OP position** in Section 1)
Hypertonic uterine action and severe pain
Hypotonic uterus, i.e. contractions start well, then slow / halt

Incoordinate uterine action
Excess moulding of fetal skull
Large caput formation
Bandl's (retraction) ring formed

Management – in pregnancy:

Obstetric referral
X-ray pelvimetry (fetal head and maternal pelvis measured on X-ray film)
Assess CPD degree – major = elective caesarean section; minor = ? trial of labour

Management – in labour:

Medical aid
Continuous fetal monitoring
Maternal condition closely monitored:
     (i) vital signs
     (ii) urine output and urinalysis
Change maternal position / mobilise
Adequate analgesia, and discontinue syntocinon if uterus hypertonic
Consider using syntocinon if uterus hypotonic
? Instrumental delivery
Emergency caesarean section if fetal / maternal compromise

Complications:

Obstructed labour
Cord prolapse
Instrumental / operative delivery
Ruptured uterus
Perinatal morbidity / death and maternal morbidity or (in developing countries) death

Student activity:

Further reading and revision of the pelvis: Bennet and Brown 2003

Changing Childbirth (DoH 1993)

A Government expert maternity group's response (chair Baroness Cumberledge) to the Winterton Report (1992), proposing radical changes in maternity services. Woman-centred, appropriate, accessible and effective care, to be facilitated by women's choices and control in care provision. Consumer satisfaction to be aided by continuity in professional care. Many units now offer a team midwifery approach to improve continuity; some offer case-load care.

Student activity:
Further reading: Page 1993; Walton and Hamilton 1995
Consider your unit's service provision in the light of *Changing Childbirth.*

Child protection

Legal protection contained in the Children Act 1989 (with consequent Rules of
Court Regulations and Guidelines) provides the framework for state and voluntary agencies to work together to prevent children suffering harm from their
carers. Local social services departments must ensure the welfare of children
when they are away from their parents – e.g. in children's homes, nurseries,
foster placements, boarding schools, or hospitals. A *Guide to Arrangements for
Inter-Agency Co-operation for the Protection of Children from Abuse* (1991) is the
'Bible' of any professional working in the field of child protection (Lyons 1995).
Hospital Trusts have local policies and guidance for child protection – e.g. for
recognition of abuse, protocols for dealing with suspected abuse, agencies to
contact, case conference procedures and record keeping. The child may be put
on the Child Protection Register or may be made the subject of a case order. The
child has a say in the proceedings.

Children Act, The 1989

Reviewed in the Adoption and Children Act 2002, the Act includes both private
and public law, e.g. what happens to children after divorce and the responsibili-
ties of the Social Service Department (SSD). Family Law Courts deal with issues
of residency following divorce, and Youth Courts with young offenders.

Main principles:
   The welfare of the child is paramount.
   Children should remain with their own families wherever possible.
   Parents retain responsibility for their children, even if no longer living with
      them.
   SSD gives appropriate help to parents of children in need.
   Children should live in a safe environment, with effective intervention if they
      are in danger.
   Children should be kept informed / participate in decisions about their future.

Cholestasis

Impaired maternal liver: a rarely diagnosed, possibly under-diagnosed condition

Aetiology:
   Unclear
   Commoner in multiple pregnancies
   ? High oestrogen levels
   ? Genetic origin

Signs and symptoms:

General pruritus (itching) in late pregnancy, often starting in hands / feet
Occasionally jaundice
Dark urine
Steatorrhoea (*ste-at-o-rea*) (undigested fat in faeces)
Raised serum bile acids / liver enzymes

Management:

Senior obstetrician referral (urgent)
Hepatologist referral
FBC; clotting screening
Prophylactic maternal vitamin K
Relieve itching locally, e.g. with calamine lotion
Induced pre-term delivery
Continuous fetal monitoring in labour
IVI *in situ*
Prepare for possible PPH

Student activity:

Further reading: Coombes 2000; McDermott 2001; Redfern and Chambers 1996; Warwick 1996

Chorionic Villus Sampling (CVS)

Not a midwife's procedure – carried out transcervically at 6–13 weeks (commonly 8–9 weeks) using ultrasound

Aim:

Aseptically remove chorionic villi (placental tissue) for investigation

Preparation:

Full explanation of procedure to woman
Consent obtained (NMC 2004a) (? counselling previously)
Dressing trolley prepared
Appropriate packs / equipment prn
Detailed scan – confirms gestation, viability, excludes multiple pregnancy

Action:

Woman made comfortable in lithotomy position
Assist by opening packs / equipment
Doctor – thoroughly cleanses thighs, vulva, cervix to minimise risk infection

Malleable cannula bent to required shape and introduced into cervical canal under USS guidance

Aspiration using a syringe / vacuum pump achieves placental biopsy

Sample placed into appropriate container, labelled, sent to laboratory

Woman made comfortable / allowed to rest until ready to go home

Advised to ring hospital if complications arise and of when results likely to be available

Procedure recorded in woman's records

Student activity:

Consider advantages / disadvantages of CVS compared to amniocentesis

CLAPA (The Cleft Lip and Palate Association)

A national support agency based in London, with local groups offering information, advice and support to parents with a baby with cleft lip and /or palate.

1st Floor, Green Man Tower   Tel. 0171 824 8110
332B Goswell Road   Fax. 020 7833 5999
London EC1V 7LQ   email info@clapa.com
   http://www.clapa.com

Clasp trial

A Collaborative Low-dose Aspirin Study in Pregnancy

Method:

A randomised, placebo, double-blind trial conducted in 213 centres in 16 countries between January 1988 and December 1992 evaluating daily low-dose aspirin in the prevention / treatment of pre-eclampsia. Over 9000 women between 12 and 32 weeks pregnant with a high risk / signs of pre-eclampsia / IUGR took part. Half had 60 mg aspirin daily, the rest a placebo (dummy). Both women and professionals were unaware which was being taken (double blind).

Results:

12% reduction in proteinuric pre-eclampsia (statistically not significant) (Every 1994).

Reduced risk of early-onset pre-eclampsia (APEC 1994)

Does not prevent IUGR (APEC 1994)

One-quarter reduced risk of severe pre-eclampsia (suggested by a meta-analysis, i.e. combining this trial with others) (APEC 1994)

Cleft lip and palate

A congenital condition, either separate or together – 'split' in upper lip; and/or in hard palate (mouth roof) or soft palate (back of mouth)

Diagnosis:

Part of the midwife's initial examination of the newborn (NB soft palate cleft easily missed)

Management:

Sensitively inform parents

Promote parent–infant attachment (distressing condition)

Paediatric and surgical referral

Aids to feeding – cup / spoon (see **cup feeding** below):

(i)   individually-made dental plate fitting roof of the baby's mouth

(ii) special teat

Repair of cleft lip usually early weeks after birth – often several operations

Repair of cleft palate when a few months old – often several operations

Referral to support group CLAPA (see above)

Student activity:

Note your local procedure for congenital cleft lip / palate

Clinical Governance

As directed in the Government White Paper *The New NHS – Modern, Dependable* (DoH 1997), Trusts have accountability for clinical governance, with practitioners accepting responsibility for developing and maintaining clinical standards. Overseeing local processes is a Commission for Health Improvement (CHIMP), while a National Institute for Clinical Excellence (NICE) gives national guidelines on services and clinical cost-effectiveness.

Student activity:

Further reading: Dimond 2000; Hart 1999

Community Health Councils (CHCs)

Independent, statutory bodies originally set up by Government in 1974, they formed a link between service providers and users, with a legal duty to represent the consumers' interests. Primary Care Trusts (PCTs) have taken over this function, and patient advisory liaison services (PALS) provide for consumer interest.

Complementary therapies

Treatment / therapy that replaces, complements, or enhances orthodox medicine.

Types:

Acupressure:
Similar to acupuncture, but using finger pressure

Acupuncture:
Traditional Chinese therapy – fine needles inserted into the skin stimulate nerve pathways, influencing other parts of the body and often offering pain relief

Aromatherapy:
Essential oils extracted from plants or flowers (neat or mixed with a base) – vapours inhaled, applied as a compress, ingested, added to bath water – e.g. aiding relaxation

Chiropractic:
Manipulation of spine

Herbalism:
Medication from plant materials – taken orally, added to the bath, applied to the skin

Homeopathy:
A holistic treatment using like to cure like – natural substances (e.g. plants, seeds, metals, insects) given orally in very dilute solutions

Hydrotherapy:
Use of water for exercise, relaxation or pain relief – e.g. aquanatal exercises and water births

Hypnotherapy:
Hypnosis, i.e. induced relaxation and auto-suggestion to control body activity or aid coping mechanism

Massage:
Rubbing and kneading of the body for relaxation or pain relief (midwives know that back rubbing relieves labour pain)

Meditation:
Deep reflection; may be accompanied by relaxation techniques

Music / sound therapy:
Soothing music aids relaxation – uterine sounds may aid baby's sleep.

Osteopathy:
Joint manipulation

Psychoprophylaxis:
Combination of breathing exercises and relaxation techniques aids coping with labour (see **relaxation techniques** below).

Physiotherapy:
Muscular exercise to improve muscle tone / joint mobility / circulation

Reflexology:
Massage of specific points in hands or feet to stimulate the energy (nerve) pathways influencing other parts of the body

Relaxation techniques (see also separate categories):
To relax mind and body

Shiatsu:
A Japanese development from Chinese medicine – simple pressure, holding techniques and gentle stretching influence nerve pathways

T.E.N.S.:
Transcutaneous (via the skin) electric nerve stimulation – low-powered electricity via small skin pads stimulates nerves, blocking pain sensations' access to cerebral cortex.

Yoga:
A Hindu method of exercise and discipline promoting physical and spiritual well-being

Dangers / contraindications in childbearing:

Joint manipulation may damage lax joints

Some herbal or aromatherapy substances are toxic / harmful to the mother / fetus

Some therapies alter BP (up or down), others uterine action (implications for progress in labour / fetal or maternal compromise)

'Emergency' conditions / situations may be missed or inappropriately managed

Professional accountability:
> A midwife must have a midwifery-appropriate qualification before practising and adhere to local policies and guidelines (NMC 2004b).
> Consider insurance (personal / vicarious) and record keeping.

Student activity:
Note your local policies on complementary therapies, aquanatal and waterbirth.
Essential reading: *Guidelines for the Administration of Medicines* (NMC 2002); *Midwives' Rules and Standards* (NMC 2004b)
Further reading: Cornwell and Dale 1995; Dimond 1998; Hodgson 1994; Kimber 1998; Tiran and Mack (eds) 1995

Confidential Enquiry into Maternal and Child Health (CEMACH)

The successor to CEMD and CESDI, launched in 2003. A self-governing body funded by the National Institute of Clinical Excellence (NICE). Enquiries will continue into maternal, perinatal and infant deaths and will be extended to encompass morbidity and a national enquiry into child health. Board of members from the Royal College of Obstetricians and Gynaecologists, Royal College of Midwives, Royal College of Paediatrics and Child Health, Royal College of Pathologists, Royal College of Anaesthetists, and Faculty of Health, with extensive lay and voluntary sector involvement.
http://www.cemach.org.uk/

Confidential Enquiry into Maternal Deaths (CEMD)

A series of triennial (3-yearly) reports that began in 1952, then covering England and Wales, but now the whole of the UK. A team of specialists audit all maternal deaths to identify causes and trends. Recommendations are often made by the team for 'best practice' in specific situations to prevent future deaths. Now an integral part of CEMACH (see above).

Confidential Enquiry into Stillbirths and Deaths in Infancy (CESDI)

Begun in 1992; data have been collected since 1993 related to infant and perinatal mortality via a rapid reporting system. Now an integral part of CEMACH (see above).

Congenital dislocation of hips

Abnormal development of one / both hip joints present at birth, with partial / complete displacement of femur head from acetabulum

Aetiology:

Approx. 1 : 1500 births

Genetic in origin – commoner in females / within families

Intrauterine position, i.e. commoner in breech / oligohydramnious cases

Diagnosis:

During routine neonatal screening (midwife / paediatrician)

Barlow's or Ortolani's test

Ultrasound scan

Management:

Paediatric referral

Orthopaedic referral

Splint to flex and abduct hips – 3 months continuous wear promotes joint formation

Complications – if undiagnosed:

Difficulty / inability walking

Leg shortening

Prolonged treatment; ? surgery

Student activity:

Note local screening method (when / by whom)

CONI (care of next infant)

A programme of support, set up by the Foundation for the Study of Infant Deaths (FSID), for families where a previous baby has died. A multidisciplinary approach is used, with local co-ordinators offering help, information, and support as required during pregnancy and following childbirth.

Contraception advice

Offered postnatally – individually timed for woman / couple's needs / wishes; cultural / religious beliefs influence acceptability.

Sexual intercourse may be commenced as soon as the mother is comfortable; caution: incidences of maternal deaths (Robinson 1998).

Keys to contraceptive advice:

Effective communication

Non-judgemental approach

Confidentiality

Offered in privacy

Up-to-date information, including availability
Timing / method acceptable to individual / couple

Methods available	*Advice*

Barrier methods:

(a) Male / female condom — Use at any time.
No-petroleum lubricant, e.g. Vaseline, in place before any genital contact.

(b) Diaphragm (cap) — Used with spermicide.
In place before any genital contact; remains in place minimum 6 hours.
Existing cap size no longer right; fit / re-fit 6 weeks PN.

(c) Spermicides – creams, gels, foam, pessaries. — Not effective alone.

Hormonal:

(a) Combined oestrogen and progesterone pill / patch — Unsuitable if breastfeeding, high BP, or smoker >35
Start 3 weeks PN – safe immediately; if later, add second method for 7 days; 12-hour safety time (if pill missed); if any later add second method for 7 days.
Pill not safe if diarrhoea, vomiting, or with use of certain antibiotics; add second method for 7 days after episode.

(b) Progesterone only (mini) pill — Suitable when combined pill is not.
Start 3 weeks PN, safe immediately.
If later start, use second method for 7 days.
3-hour safety time if pill missed – if any later, use second method for 7 days.
Not safe if diarrhoea, vomiting; add second method for 7 days after episode.
Unaffected by antibiotics.

(c) Progesterone, IM (slow release) — ? Delayed return of fertility
? Menstrual irregularities
Start 5th day PN, safe immediately.
Start after 6 weeks if BF, and also use second method for 7 days.
Repeat every 12 weeks (Depo-Provera).
Repeat every 8 weeks (Noristat).

(d) Progesterone implants:	1 capsule implanted under skin (Implanon) of upper arm (slow release).
	Insert 21 days PN; safe immediately.
	If inserted any later, also use second method for 7 days.
	Replace 5-yearly.
(e) Progesterone intrauterine system (e.g. Mirena) (slow release)	Hormone-impregnated coil.
	Insert 6 weeks PN, safe immediately.
	Replace 3-yearly.

Intrauterine contraceptive device (IUCD) (coil):

Insert 6 weeks PN; safe immediately.
Replace 3–5-yearly.
First 2–3 periods ? heavy / painful.

Natural family planning:

Acceptable in certain religions / cultures.
Needs knowledge / motivation.
Needs specialist teaching.

Emergency contraception:

After unprotected intercourse / failed contraceptive method.

(a) Hormonal (Schering PC4)	High progesterone tabs. within 72 hours.
	Available from family planning clinics, GP, some A and E departments, pregnancy advisory clinics and pharmacists.
(b) IUCD	Inserted within 5 days after intercourse or within 5 days after ovulation.
	Available family planning clinics, some GPs.

Sterilisation:

(a) Female tubal ligation	Usually after 12 weeks PN.
	General anaesthetic / hospital stay.
	Safe immediately.
	NHS / private hospital.
(b) Male vasectomy	Performed at any time.
	Unsafe until 3 semen specimens sperm-free – may take several weeks.
	Local / general anaesthetic – day case NHS (waiting list) / private hospital.
? Future	male 'pill' – under development

Student activity:

Identify local family planning clinics – times and locations
Consider the needs of teenagers, specific religious / ethnic groups

Further reading: Dimond 2002 Chapter 10; Harden 1999; Kelly 1999; Kirsten *et al.* 1999; Norman 1995; Silverstone 1997; Urwin 1995; Waugh 2000

Convulsions – see **eclampsia**; **epilepsy**; **jittery baby** below

Cord prolapse / presentation

Prolapse – cord loop presents following membrane rupture

Presentation – cord loop lies below presenting part, membranes intact (occult if unseen/felt at side)

Aetiology:

Long cord increases risk

Poorly fitting presenting part in maternal pelvis, e.g.:

    (i)   malpresentation – e.g. breech (especially footling); shoulder

    (ii)   malposition, e.g. occipito-posterior

    (iii)   small fetus, e.g. pre-term labour

    (iv)   high presenting part – especially at membrane rupture

    (v)   CPD, e.g. abnormal maternal pelvis; large baby

    (vi)   multiple pregnancy

    (vii) uterine fibroids

    (viii) placenta praevia

Diagnosis:

Pregnancy – USS

Labour:

    (i)   VE

    (ii) suspected in certain CTG patterns

Management (see Figures 3.1, 3.2 on pp. 70, 71):

Complications:

Fetal hypoxia due to:

    (i)   cord compression

    (ii) vessel spasm from cooling / drying / handling

Birth asphyxia

Long-term consequences of hypoxia / asphyxia

Perinatal death

Surgical intervention for mother – immediate / long-term risks

Psychological trauma / post-traumatic stress

Student activity:

Note your local policy / procedures

Further reading: Prabulos and Philipson 1998; Saunders 1997; Squire 2002

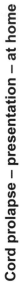

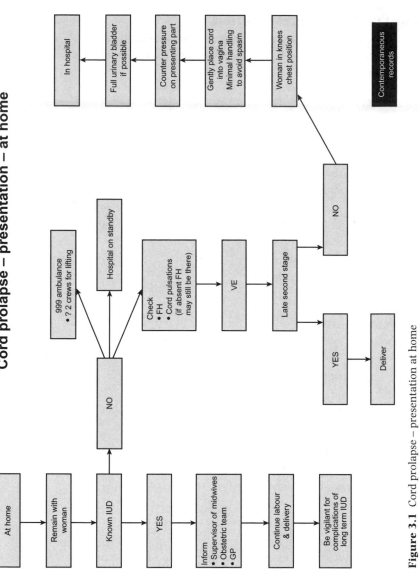

Figure 3.1 Cord prolapse – presentation at home

Cord prolapse – presentation – in hospital

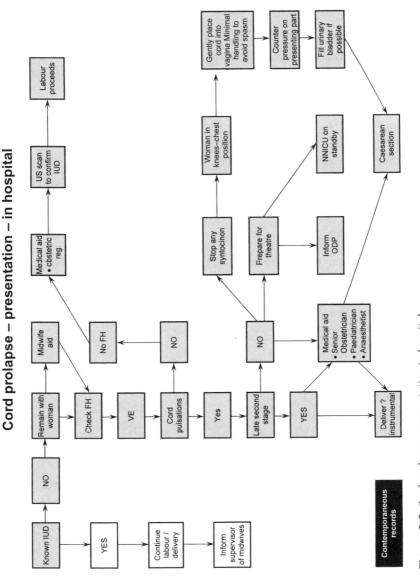

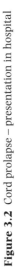

Figure 3.2 Cord prolapse – presentation in hospital

Cramp
Painful muscle spasms – usually legs

Aetiology:
common in pregnancy – cause unproven

Management:
Massage and dorsiflexion of leg (pointing toes towards knee)

Crying baby
Causes:
Hunger
Pain – wind; colic; trauma; illness
Wrong temperature – too hot / cold
Uncomfortable – position; soiled nappy
Lonely; frightened; bored; startled

Management:
Identify cause:
? Obvious – feed time / rooting reflex; known trauma / illness
Thorough history from mother / records

Observe baby's:
General well-being / condition:
  (i)   urine output
  (ii) stool colour, consistency, frequency
  (iii) skin colour / tone
General behaviour:
  (i)   state of alertness
  (ii) rapid leg movements ? indicate wind / colic
  (iii) cry type – shrill sound ? cerebral irritation / pain
  (iv) cry onset – sudden noise; dark / quiet ? fear / loneliness
  (v)   cry ceasing – when spoken to / nursed (relieves boredom)
  (vi) eagerness to feed
Environment :
  (i)   clothing / bedding
  (ii) room temperature

Thorough examination:
Temperature and heart rate
State of fontanelle
Muscle tone and reflexes

Consider:
> Feed type, frequency, amount
> Breastfeeding mother's fluid / nutritional intake
> Correct preparation, storage, feeding technique of formula

Provide:
> Appropriate information / advice
> Promotion mother's confidence – encouragement / support
> Medical aid prn

Cultural aspects related to childbirth

Culture – a way of life (values, beliefs, conduct). Reproduction, menstruation, fertility and sexuality are sensitive issues surrounded by customs, religious practices, folk beliefs, taboos. Pregnancy / parenthood may have many different meanings – you do not have to share other people's beliefs to provide care sympathetically. These points are a *guide* only, as everyone is individual and may not follow these customs. Always ask what the individual wishes. Non-British naming systems may present difficulties in addressing individuals and record-keeping.

Pregnancy:
> A transition period – often viewed as dangerous
> Modesty may make examination difficult / only acceptable by another woman.
> Woman may be accompanied by husband or son, only communicating through him (not just a language problem).
> Husband's permission may have to be sought before treatment / care given.
> Rules may govern workload during pregnancy – often reduced or stopped by specific weeks.

Childbirth:
> May be viewed as natural, supernatural, a duty, an illness, a normal physiological process, a private or social event, a sexual experience.
> In biblical times associated with punishment for sins of Eve; therefore pain and sorrow essential.
> Choice of analgesia and expression of pain may be culturally determined (Queen Victoria's use of chloroform in 1853 for a pain-free labour initiated acceptance of pain relief for labour in the UK).

Menstruation and the postnatal period:
> Women may be viewed as unclean, dangerous, polluting, magical, spiritual, powerful;

they may be isolated physically, with certain restrictions, e.g. no hair-washing,
swimming, sexual contact / physical contact with men.

Rules on bed rest / confinement; diet; re-introduction to family; ritual cleansing
(i.e. physically and spiritually)

Social status may be changed.

Rules on return to work may apply.

Fetal / baby's rights:

Stage of attainment of human status varies – this influences rules re:

     (i)   abortion

     (ii) stillbirth burial

     (iii) infant naming

     (iv) infant-rearing practices

Ceremonies for baby:

Bathing may / may not be acceptable

Circumcision

Naming – several days / months later

Baptism

Specific rules for stillbirth, e.g. who can touch the baby, disposal of the body,
agreement to post-mortem

Infant feeding:

Method of feeding may have social, symbolic or economic meaning.

Breastfeeding may be delayed until all colostrum expressed (seen as poison).

Breastfeeding may be acceptable in public or only privately.

Dietary rules on what can be eaten may apply during breastfeeding.

Role of men:

Varies from total avoidance / physical contact, to close intimacy.

New Guinea husbands must 'build' the fetus and 'feed' the uterus with semen.

Presence at delivery ranges from taboo to expected.

Ritual *couvade* – men go through sympathetic labour in another place.

Chinese culture, diet / rituals

May be Christian, Muslim or Buddhist.

Good manners and politeness important.

Woman may wish female professional.

Open declaration of emotion may not be acceptable; may express social or psychological problems as physical symptoms, e.g. pain in an organ (NB danger
that depression is missed or mis-diagnosed).

Believe in balance of *Yin* (cold principle) and *Yang* (hot principle) by use of appropriate food or medication – meat, eggs, rice wine, gaseous drinks, spicy foods, iron and vitamin tablets are 'hot'; bland, low-fat foods, vegetables, fruit, milk and milk products are cold; rice, fish and noodles are neutral.

Some illnesses / conditions are hot, e.g. pregnancy, or cold, e.g. menstruation and puerperium.

Postnatally isolated in one room, unable to eat with the family, or wash hair, dishes or clothes; cold water / wind, e.g. fan or open window, to be avoided.

Baby's 'hot' or 'cold' condition influences maternal diet when breastfeeding.

Baby not bathed for three days.

Official birth celebration at one month.

Hindu culture, diet / rituals

Avoid meat, especially beef; eggs may / not be eaten (implications for medicines).

Caste system (social class) strictly recognised.

Relatives visit for prayer within 4 days of birth.

40 days postnatal rest.

Jehovah's Witness – beliefs

A Christian group who believe, for Bible-based reasons, that they must refuse blood or blood products, e.g. plasma (alternatives acceptable); anti D immunoglobulin. Possible difficulties when APH or PPH occurs (see the Annexe to Chapter 3 in Hibbard *et al.* 1996), or in Rhesus-negative women.

Jewish – diet / rituals

Food must be *Kosher*, i.e. specifically prepared, ritually accepted; no pork / shellfish.

Sabbath (dusk Friday to dusk Saturday) restricts activities, e.g. switching on light.

Women modest, ? inform children / family of pregnancy (no AN home visit – confidentiality).

Husband may sit in labour room / near by, reading prayers: no physical contact.

Bed rest taken for 10 days postnatally (NB prevention of DVT).

Postnatally / during menstruation (unclean) – for set time husbands avoid physical contact.

Breastfeeding is the norm.

Male circumcision by a highly trained expert (may be a Rabbi) on the 8th day.

Muslim culture, diet / rituals

Follow religion of Islam.

Food *Halal*, i.e. specifically prepared, i.e. lawful / permitted; honey and dried prunes religious food; no pork or alcohol (implications for medication).

Ramadan (1 month of fasting from dawn to dusk): diabetics and breastfeeding women are exempt, but pregnant women are not (they may not comply).

May not discuss intimate topics through husband or son when acting as interpreter.

Modesty may mean a female professional must attend.

Pain of labour accepted without analgesia.

All male babies circumcised.

Baby's head shaved at birth / within 14 days.

Colostrum may be expressed and not given to baby.

A call to prayer whispered into baby's ear by father / religious person soon after birth.

Outward grief suppressed if stillbirth.

Sikh culture, rituals / diet

No beef, possibly vegetarian (implications for some medication).

Women comparatively outgoing / ? woman doctor.

40 days postnatal rest.

Student activity:

Further reading: Bharj 1995; Chan 1995; Chesney 1995; Cheung 1996a, 1996b; Hennings *et al.* 1996; Schott and Henley 1996; Waterhouse 1994; Zaidi 1994

Cup feeding

Aim:

Provide an alternative method of giving breast milk (or formula milk) to babies who are unable or too weak / immature to suck

Preparation:

Expressed breast milk / formula milk in sterile container

Explain procedure to mother

Baby clean / comfortable

Sterile medicine cup (or similar) for giving feed

Feeding chart labelled

Action:

Hold baby securely – upright position, maintaining eye contact.

Place a few ml of milk into cup.

Place the cup just touching lower lip; tip it, allowing baby to lap milk with its tongue.

Leaving cup in position during the feed allows baby to control own intake.

Observe baby carefully, ensuring no problems swallowing.

Refill cup prn, noting amount taken each time.

Allow plenty of time for feed.

Following feed, settle baby comfortably.

Record intake accurately on feeding chart.

Wash cup thoroughly prior to re-sterilising it.

Student activity:
Further reading: Lang 1994

Cystitis
Bladder inflammation – untreated ? progress to severe UTI / septicaemia

Aetiology:
Commonly bacterial, often *E. coli* organism (normal bowel flora)

Signs and symptoms:
Stinging / burning on micturition (PU)

Lower abdominal discomfort / pain

Pyrexia (high temperature)

General malaise (feel unwell)

Investigations:
see **urinary tract infection – UTI** in Section 2

Management:
Copious oral fluids

Appropriate medication

Good hygiene minimises recurrence.

Tissue cleansing from front to back avoids anal contamination.

Regular / complete bladder emptying (problematic during pregnancy)

Emptying bladder following sexual intercourse

Deep vein thrombosis (also see **embolism** below)
Thrombosis (clot formation) in a deep vein – commonly lower leg; iliac or femoral veins

Risk factors:
Immobility, e.g. bed rest; operative delivery

Previous history of thromboembolic disorder

Obesity

Smoking

Increases with age

Prevention:

Avoid immobility – during labour / postnatally

Anticoagulants – e.g. heparin – if major risk (Lewis 1998; Drife in Lewis 2004,
   p. 61)

TED stockings (see Section 1) if identified risk

Avoid dehydration

No oestrogen, as in e.g. combined oral contraception

Signs and symptoms:

? Asymptomatic

Slight pyrexia / slight tachycardia

Lower abdominal; groin; calf pain, depending on clot location

Leg ? oedematous, pale, cooler

Diagnosis:

History

Clot location by USS / venography (X-ray following injection of dye into
   veins)

Management:

See Drife in Lewis 2001, p. 49

Medical aid

Anticoagulants – IV heparin – bolus dose and / or in an intravenous infusion,
   or SC heparin

Blood for clotting screening

Bed rest – ? elevate foot of bed; use a bed cradle

Analgesics

Observe for abnormal bleeding, e.g. lochia / wounds; general condition; vital
   signs

Anticoagulants continued after discharge – usually orally, i.e. heparin in pregnancy / warfarin postnatal

Complications:

Potentially life-threatening – moving clot (embolism) lodges elsewhere – commonly lung (pulmonary embolism) or brain (cerebral embolism)

Thromboembolic conditions are the highest cause of direct maternal deaths in
   UK (Lewis 2004).

Delivery technique

As independent, accountable practitioners, midwives develop individual views on childbirth management. Partnership in care / choices in position for birth means that prescriptive delivery techniques are no longer feasible. However, principles of safe delivery that apply for home and hospital are included here.

Aim:

Deliver the baby safely.

Minimise harm to both mother / baby.

Early detection / management of deviations from normal.

Reduce the risk of postnatal infection.

Accommodate woman's / partner's wishes in achieving a satisfactory / fulfilling outcome.

Preparation:

Vaginal delivery can only be a clean (rather than an aseptic) procedure; however:

All preparations as for aseptic technique

Delivery pack / instruments

Cleansing solution (note local policy) – warmed if possible

Syntometrine prepared for IM injection prn

Ensure warm environment / cot

Identification bands for newborn in hospital – (see **identification of newborn at birth** below)

Other equipment to aid woman's choice of position – e.g. wedges, bean bags, cushions

Discussion with woman previously about any special wishes, e.g. partner to cut cord

Position yourself on mother's right (depending on birth position adopted).

Action:

Directed pushing (Valsalva manoeuvre) unnecessary in the light of research; however, woman may value midwife's instruction, particularly as head is crowning.

Spontaneous pushing encouraged

Delivery pack opened / equipment prepared once progress being made (timing depends on parity / position)

Sterile gloves / protective clothing worn

Vulva / perineum swabbed, drapes on bed / floor (depends on birth position)

Delivery of head in occipito-anterior position:

Allow head to advance with maternal effort

As head distends perineum apply pressure with left cupped hand to prevent rapid delivery / perineal trauma (see **HOOP Study** below) (flexing the head of doubtful value)

As the head crowns, woman asked not to push but pant / breathe Entonox to facilitate slow delivery

Once the biparietal diameter has delivered, head is eased out by extension.

Whilst awaiting restitution / external rotation, feel neck for cord

If cord present and loose – a loop can be freed by pulling over the head

If the cord present and very tight, apply two artery forceps and cut between – loosen from around the neck.

When the shoulders have rotated, encourage woman to push with the next contraction – midwife guides the baby's head towards the perineum, allowing delivery of anterior shoulder.

Syntometrine commonly given by an assistant at this point.

Baby's head is eased towards the symphysis, releasing posterior shoulder

Baby is supported beneath the axillae; body delivered towards mother's abdomen (NB check that direct skin-to-skin contact is acceptable).

Apgar score is assessed.

Cord commonly cut at this point (but see **delivery** – third-stage management below).

Dry baby and observe onset of respirations.

Mother baby skin-to-skin contact (Sheridan 1999; Finigan and Davies 2004) or wrap in a warm towel for mother to hold.

Apgar score

SIGN	0	1	2	SCORE
Colour (appearance)	Pale / blue	Pink with blue extremities	Completely pink	
Apex beat (pulse)	Absent	Slow - less than 100	More than 100	
Response to stimuli (grimace)	No response	Facial grimace	Crying	
Muscle activity	Limp	Some flexion of limbs	Active movements	
Respiratory effort	Absent	Slow irregular cry	Strong cry	
			TOTAL SCORE	

Figure 4 Apgar score

Third-stage management (see Figures 5.1, 5.2, on pp. 82–3):
>   (i)   usually controlled cord traction (CCT) or modified Brandt–Andrews
>   (ii) physiological at mother's informed request
>   (iii) Brandt–Andrews method (rarely used now).

Perineum / vagina / cervix examined to assess any trauma

Placenta / membranes checked for completeness (see **placental examination** below)

Blood loss estimated

Routine observations – vital signs

Uterus palpated to ensure good contraction

Make mother comfortable

Baby's top-to-toe examination (with mother) if satisfactory condition

Apply ID bands in hospital setting (see **identification of newborn** below)

Baby put to the breast prn

Mother, partner, baby left for private time together (if condition allows)

Contemporaneous records completed

After approximately one hour, mother / baby transferred to postnatal area.

Delivery of head in persistent occipito-posterior (OP) position (face-to-pubes) (see Diagrams 2.1, 2.2, 2.3 on pp. 86–7):

Occurs after short rotation in OP position

Head is usually deflexed – wider engaging diameter

Increased risk of perineal trauma / ? episiotomy

Consider squatting position – increases diameters of pelvic outlet

All-fours / kneeling position ? relieves backache associated with OP position.

Sinciput leading part – flexion of the fetal head is encouraged by exerting pressure with the fingers of the left hand towards the symphysis.

When the occiput sweeps the perineum the head extended slightly to release baby's glabella and face.

Remainder of the delivery conducted as previously.

Delivery of a face presentation (see Diagrams 1.1, 1.2, 1.3 on pp. 84–5):

May be primary presentation or, more commonly, secondary.

Associated with OP position – wider diameter delayed at pelvic brim, head completely extends, becoming mento-anterior position.

(NB mento-posterior position will not deliver vaginally – insufficient pelvic space for occiput anteriorly.)

VEs kept to a minimum / performed very carefully during the first stage of labour – preventing tissues damage.

Management of third stage of labour – physiological and active

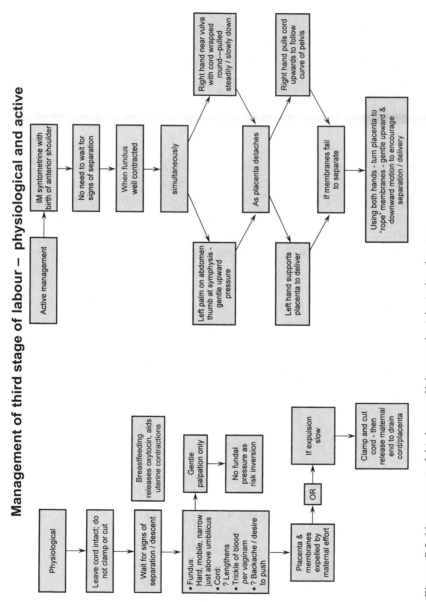

Figure 5.1 Management of third stage of labour – physiological and active

Management of third stage – alternative active management

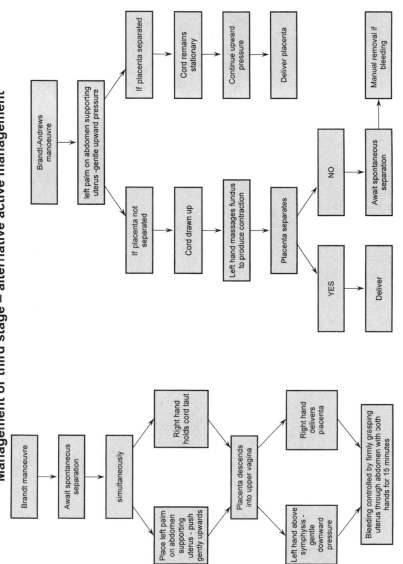

Figure 5.2 Management of third stage of labour – alternative active management

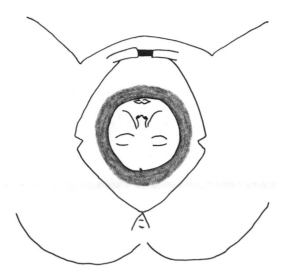

Face presentation:
Diagram 1.1 Landmarks on vaginal examination:
  Orbital ridges
  Nose
  Cheek bones
  Mouth

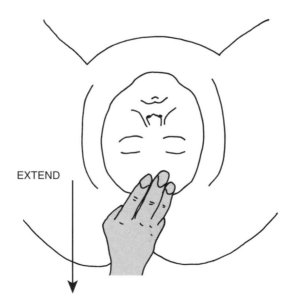

EXTEND

Diagram 1.2 Delivery of the head:
  Extend the head further to allow delivery of the chin from under the pubic arch

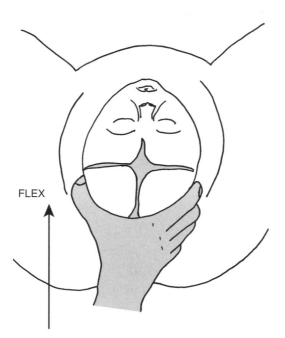

FLEX

Diagram 1.3 When the chin is released, flex the head to allow the occiput to sweep the perineum

Considerable pressure to face from pelvic floor during descent through the birth canal – ? tissues damage – bruised / oedematous (inform woman / partner)

Paediatrician present at the delivery – ? problems with resuscitation

Action:

Episiotomy necessary to prevent perineal trauma.

Maintain gentle pressure on sinciput allowing mentum to deliver first under pubic arch.

Sinciput, vertex, occiput delivered by flexion.

Avoid facial trauma whilst feeling round the neck for cord.

Continue as normal delivery – pass baby to paediatrician for examination / resuscitation.

NB – baby may have head retraction for a few days following delivery – ? severe bruising causing feeding problems / re-absorption jaundice – ? observe / manage in SCBU.

Student activity:

Revise mechanisms of labour.

Further reading: HOOP Study; McCandlish 1999; McCandlish *et al.* 1998; Parnell *et al.* 1993; Thomson 1993b, 1995

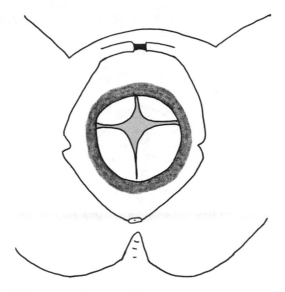

Persistent occipito-posterior position:

Diagram 2.1 Landmarks on vaginal examination:
  Anterior fontanelle
  Sagittal suture
  Parietal bones

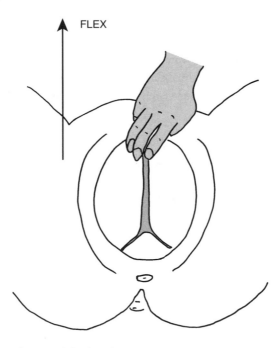

FLEX

Diagram 2.2 Delivery of the head:
  Flex the head towards the symphysis pubis if deflexed as this allows the smaller
    diameter to come through the introitus
  Allow the occiput to sweep the perineum

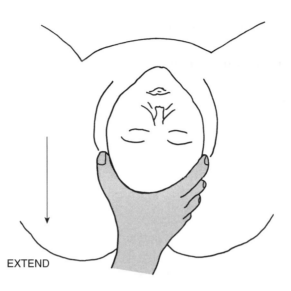

EXTEND

Diagram 2.3 When the occiput has been delivered, extend the head to bring the face under the sub-pubic arch and allow the chin to escape

Diabetes mellitus

Type I diabetes:

Pancreatic function is poor / non-existent.

Daily insulin by subcutaneous injection is required.

More common in younger people.

Type II diabetes:

Some pancreatic function remains.

Oral medications either stimulate insulin production or aid glucose utilisation.

Onset commoner in older people.

Impaired glucose tolerance (latent diabetes):

Insulin adequate but glucose metabolism inefficient.

Occurs only at times of stress.

May develop into frank diabetes in later life.

Gestational diabetes:

Occurs only during pregnancy (2%–5% pregnancies).

Resolves following childbirth.

May develop into frank diabetes in later life.

Aetiology – gestational diabetes

Remains uncertain; often unrecognised.

Generally presents in the 3rd trimester.

Linked to raised placental hormones.

May be due to:

    (i)   inadequate insulin production for increased needs

    (ii) abnormal carbohydrate metabolism

    (iii) insulin resistance.

Women at greatest risk:

    (i)   ethnic groups

    (ii) older women

    (iii) family history of diabetes

    (iv) previous history of gestational diabetes

    (v)   previous large baby

    (vi) previous unexplained stillbirth / neonatal death.

Diagnosis:

Random blood glucose if 1+ or more of glucose on dip stick

Fasting blood glucose >6 mmol / l (lab. test) – ? glucose tolerance test needed (GTT)

Non-fasting blood glucose >7 mmol / l (lab. test) – ? GTT

GTT – 2 hours after 75 g oral glucose:

    (i)   blood glucose levels >8 mmol / l = gestational diabetes.

    (ii) blood glucose levels 6–8 mmol / l = impaired glucose tolerance.

Diabetes and pregnancy

Pre-conception:

Sub-fertility if poor control.

Identify severity of diabetic changes, i.e. nephropathy; neuropathy; retinopathy (kidney; nerve; eye).

Discuss risks of worsening of complications, ? avoid pregnancy (informed choice).

Treat complications.

'Tight' control of blood glucose levels (5–6 mmol / l) improves pregnancy outcome.

Type II diabetics: change to insulin.

Care from diabetes specialist consultant and nurse.

Dietary advice from dietitian; includes folic acid 4 mg daily.

Pregnancy:

Insulin requirements increase from 20 weeks.

Insulin dose / frequency may need changing.

Diabetic complications, especially retinopathy, may worsen.

Hypoglycaemic attacks may increase with 'tight' control.

Continue 'tight' control on blood glucose levels (5.5–6.0 mmol / l fasting) by dietary control and exercise.

Insulin – but hypoglycaemic attacks more likely and glucagon IM provided and partner / family instructed when and how to administer.

Increase blood glucose monitoring (urinary glucose unreliable).

Strategies for coping with morning sickness.

Close liaison with diabetes specialists throughout pregnancy.

Early recognition / treatment of retinopathy.

Gestational diabetes:

Rapid specialist referral if suspected / diagnosed.

Dietary advice / weight reduction

Insulin regime as indicated

Pregnancy and diabetes

Increased risk of complications, particularly when control poor, e.g.

Maternal:

Infection:

    (i)   UTI

    (ii) vulvo-vaginitis, especially *Monilia* (thrush)

    (iii) puerperal sepsis

Cardiovascular:

    (i)   PPH risk (if polyhydramnios)

    (ii) PIH, pre-eclampsia, eclampsia risk

    (iii) proteinuria and oedema likely

    (iv) thromboembolic disorders risk

Genital tract trauma due to large baby with possible long-term consequences

Baby:

Abortion

    (i)   spontaneous / induced

    (ii) higher incidence often linked to fetal abnormalities

Pre-term delivery

    (i)   induced

    (ii) spontaneous

    (iii) caesarean section

Oligohydramnios – associated with

    (i)   large baby

    (ii) large placenta

    (iii) pre-term labour

    (iv) congenital abnormalities:

        (a) cardiovascular

        (b) renal

        (c) central nervous system, e.g. anencephaly

        (d) caudal regression syndrome, i.e. sacral ageneses and lower-limb hypoplasia

        (e) skeletal

        (f) hypospadias (urethral opening on underside of penis)

IUD – increased risk in last 3–4 weeks – associated with:

    (i)   high maternal glycosylated haemoglobin (HbA$_1$C) reducing O$_2$ transfer across placenta

    (ii) maternal ketoacidosis

    (iii) maternal infection

    (iv) hypertensive disorders

IUGR – due to:

    (i)   poor uterine perfusion / placental insufficiency

    (ii) fetal malformations

    (iii) maternal infection

    (iv) maternal hypertensive disorders

Fetal distress in labour – due to:

    (i)   placental insufficiency

    (ii) maternal ketoacidosis

    (iii) prolonged labour

    (iv) shoulder dystocia

Macrosomia – i.e. baby >4000 g (diabetic cherub) – risk of:

    (i)   perinatal / neonatal death

    (ii) prolonged labour

    (iii) shoulder dystocia

    (iv) birth injury

    (v) birth asphyxia

    (vi) instrumental / operative delivery

RDS (neonatal) – due to:

    (i)   high fetal insulin inhibiting surfactant production

    (ii) prematurity

Hypoglycaemia (neonatal) – blood glucose level <2.5 mmol / l (or lower – controversial) occurs 1–1½ hours later, caused by fetal hyperinsulinaemia.

Polycythaemia (excess rbc) hyperviscosity (sticky blood) due to:

    high maternal glycosylated haemoglobin (HbA$_1$C), reducing O$_2$ transfer across placenta, causes plethora (redness).

Cardiovascular disorders and tachycardia

(i) tachypnoea (rapid breathing) and respiratory distress

(ii) convulsions

Hypocalcaemia (low calcium) – 2–3 days after birth

(i) increased muscle tone; twitching; convulsions

(ii) associated with respiratory distress; asphyxia; acidosis.

Jaundice – 2–3 days after birth, due to:

(i) increased haemolysis of rbc (polycythaemia)

(ii) inhibited liver enzymes

(iii) prematurity

Infection – more prone

Long-term outcome:

(i) higher incidence of obesity

(ii) increased incidence of diabetes.

Management – pregnancy

Multi-professional team approach, ideally combined appointments

Early antenatal booking

Obstetric consultant to lead care

? Some community-based midwife care (depending on condition)

Discuss plan of care with woman

Regular ultrasound scans / biophysical profiles:

Date pregnancy

Identify abnormalities

Monitor fetal well-being

Blood monitoring:

glycosylated haemoglobin (HbA$_1$C) – venous blood

reagent strip with a meter at home – peripheral blood

Early recognition / management of PIH / pre-eclampsia

Early recognition / treatment of infections, especially UTI

Hospitalisation for complications

? Estimation fetal lung maturity 37–38 weeks (rarely amniocentesis / LS ratio)

Consider optimal delivery time – often 38 weeks – no consensus (CESDI 1999)

Consider appropriate labour management, i.e. spontaneous / induced and delivery mode, i.e. normal or elective caesarean section

Management – labour:

Senior obstetrician, anaesthetist, diabetes specialist involved.

Experienced midwife supervising.

Usual labour management – vigilant for complications.

Analgesia prn – ? epidural beneficial

Clear fluids only orally.

IVI 10% glucose / dextrose at 10 g per hour (i.e. 100 ml / hour) = less fluid overload than 5% glucose

IV insulin (using pump) according to blood glucose levels

Peripheral blood glucose levels hourly using a reagent strip and meter

Urinalysis for ketones

? Continuous electronic monitoring

? Fetal blood sampling – early identification of fetal compromise

Pre-term labour – maternal IM corticosteroids (observe for hyperglycaemia and ketoacidosis)

Paediatrician at delivery

Neonatal unit on standby

Emergency caesarean section if doubt about vaginal delivery.

Management – postnatal:

Insulin requirements fall rapidly after delivery:
- (i)   halve insulin infusion immediately after 3rd stage
- (ii) return to pre-pregnant insulin as soon as normal diet taken.

Blood glucose monitoring continues.

Urinary glucose levels more reliable.

Prophylactic antibiotics following caesarean section.

Breastfeeding encouraged (increased carbohydrate without insulin increase).

6 week postnatal appointment

Referral to diabetes clinic for follow-up

GTT at 3 months for gestational diabetics / advise long-term follow-up (risk of late-onset diabetes)

Pre-conception advice may be appropriate.

Contraception – ? IUCD (infection risk); oral; barrier methods

Management – neonate:

Information / support parents

Baby with mother unless special care needed

Hypoglycaemia:

Monitor blood glucose (see **heel prick** below)
- (i)   HemoCue™ system (more accurate for low levels of glucose than reagent strip and meter)
- (ii) ideally, true blood glucose (TBG) on venous blood.

Early feeding

Neonatal unit if symptomatic; IVI glucose

RDS:
  Neonatal unit
  Surfactant administered.

Polycythaemia and hyperviscosity:
  Early clamping of cord to prevent excess blood transfer
  NNU if symptomatic
  Exchange blood-for-plasma transfusion

Hypocalcaemia:
  Monitor blood levels
  IM or IV calcium

Jaundice:
  Usual management

Infection:
  Early recognition and treatment

SGA / prematurity:
  Usual management

Abnormalities:
  Individualised management

Student activity:
Revise anatomy and physiology of the pancreas (see Roberts 1996)
Revise signs, symptoms, diagnosis of diabetes
Familiarise yourself with all types of insulin / administration
Note your local policy and procedures for:
        (i)   screening for gestational diabetes
        (ii) care of the diabetic woman during pregnancy, labour and
              puerperium
        (iii) neonatal care.
Further reading: Casson *et al.* 1997; Cowan 1997; Simmons 1997; Turner 1999b;
    Watkins 1998; Young 1997

Disseminated intravascular coagulation (coagulopathy) (DIC)

Disseminated = throughout the body; intravascular = within the blood vessels;
    coagulation = clotting.

Aetiology:

A syndrome (secondary to primary event)

Widespread clot formation causes abnormal fibrinogen and clotting factor consumption – clotting mechanism fails – haemorrhage occurs

Primary event:

Severe tissue damage

APH / PPH

Amniotic fluid embolism

Severe pre-eclampsia / eclampsia

Prolonged IUD (intrauterine death)

Septicaemia

Inherited coagulation disorder

Low platelets

Prevention:

Prevent, treat, manage primary event

Coagulation defect screening / abnormalities aggressively managed

Management – initial (see Figure 6, p. 95):

Management – subsequent:

Postnatal debriefing and psychological support

Complications:

Maternal death

Sheehan's syndrome

Renal failure

Infection risk increased

Psychological morbidity, e.g. post-traumatic stress (see **postnatal depression** below)

Student activity:

Note your local policy / procedures for DIC.

Familiarise yourself with intensive care charts/records.

Down's Syndrome

A genetic abnormality of chromosome 21, either trisomy (i.e. 3 instead of 2 chromosomes) or a translocation of a piece of one of the chromosomes on to another.

See **antenatal screening** in Section 2 above.

Disseminated intravascular coagulation (DIC)

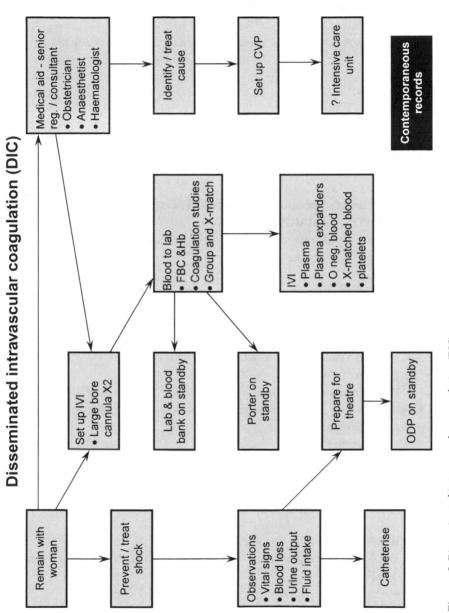

Figure 6 Disseminated intravascular coagulation (DIC)

Down's Syndrome Association – offer information and support to parents and professionals.

Langdown Down Centre	Tel. 0845 230 0372
2a Langdown Park,	Fax. 0845 230 0373
Teddington, TW11 9PS	email info@downs-syndrome.org.uk
	http://www.downs-syndrome.org.uk

Student activity:
Further reading: Tolliss 1995

Drug-addicted mother and neonate
– see **substance-abusing mother and baby** and **smoking in pregnancy** below

Eclampsia (see also **pregnancy-induced hypertension (PIH) and pre-eclampsia** below; and **MAGPIE trial** below)
Fitting (like major epileptic fits) associated with childbearing – during pregnancy, labour or first 72 hours postnatally

Signs and symptoms:
? Evidence of pre-eclampsia / PIH

Mother may 'feel strange'

Premonitory stage – eyes may roll, mild facial and / or hand tremors

Tonic stage – spasmodic muscle activity up to 30 seconds

    (i)   clenched teeth / fists

    (ii) respirations stop = cyanosis

Clonic stage – jerky / violent muscle movements may last 2 minutes

    (i)   frothy saliva

    (ii) may bite tongue

    (iii) may inhale mucus / vomit

Coma – deep unconsciousness – last minutes / hours – cyanosis fades

Management (see Figure 7, p. 97):

Prevention:
Early and prompt treatment of pre-eclampsia (see **MAGPIE trial** and Lewis 2001 p. 76)

End the pregnancy – ? caesarean section

Consequences:
Status eclampticus, i.e. continual fitting – increases risks

Maternal / infant morbidity

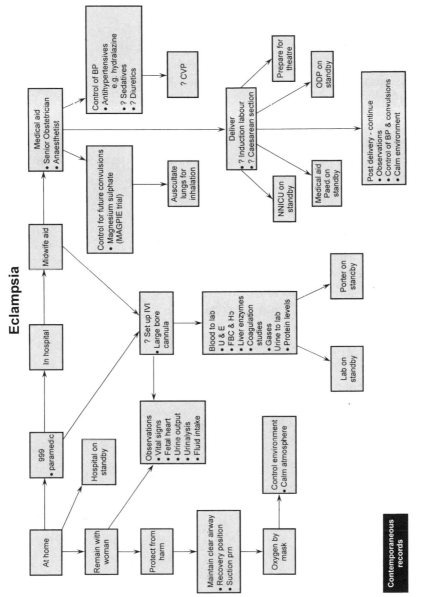

Figure 7 Eclampsia

Maternal death
    5 cases between 1997 and 1999 (Lewis 2001)
    6 cases between 2000 and 2002 (Lewis 2004)
Perinatal death (intrauterine hypoxia)

Student activity:
Compare / contrast eclampsia / epileptic seizure
Further reading: Draycott *et al.* 2000; Duley 1995; Duley *et al.* 2003; Sibai 2005

Embolism
A moved clot of blood that commonly lodges in the lung (pulmonary – PE) or in the brain (cerebral), frequently having arisen from a DVT.

Cerebral thrombosis – signs and symptoms:
Sudden collapse / death / unconsciousness
Severe headache / pain
Signs of cerebro-vascular accident (CVA = stroke), e.g.
        (i)   paralysis (limb, facial)
        (ii) dysphasia (difficulty speaking)

Cerebral thrombosis – diagnosis:
History
CAT scan confirms

Pulmonary embolism – signs and symptoms:

Mild	*Severe*
slight pyrexia	obvious pyrexia
slight dyspnoea (difficulty breathing)	severe dyspnoea
slight transient chest pain	severe chest pain
raised respiration rate	cyanosis
unproductive cough	haemoptysis (coughing up blood)
	respiratory arrest
	death

Pulmonary embolism – diagnosis:
History
Chest X-ray / scan

Management:
    Resuscitation prn
    Medical aid – obstetric team, physicians, anaesthetists
    Anticoagulants
    IVI
    Psychological support to mother, partner, family

Complications:
    Death – thromboembolism is the commonest cause of maternal mortality in
        the UK (Lewis 2004)
    Long-term morbidity from respiratory damage
    Long-term morbidity from paralysis
    Psychological morbidity
    Psycho-social effects on family

Student activity:
Further reading: Lewis 2004, http://www.cemach.org.uk

Epigastric pain
Pain in the upper abdomen / lower chest behind sternum

Aetiology:
    Heartburn, dyspepsia (indigestion), wind (see **heartburn** below)
    Oesophagitis (inflamed oesophagus due to acid reflux)
    Bleeding under liver capsule in severe (fulminating) pre-eclampsia, often before
        eclampsia

Management:
    Differential diagnosis vital
    Indigestion, wind, oesophagitis – antacids (see Jones 1999)
    Pre-eclampsia / eclampsia (see **eclampsia** in Section 2 above and **pregnancy-
        induced hypertension/pre-eclampsia** below)

Epilepsy
Abnormal brain electrical impulses

Types:
Clinical seizure type and EEG findings denote classification – but is not always
    clear-cut

Generalised seizures may:

Be convulsive / not

Involve jerking muscle movements (myoclonic)

Involve body / limbs stiffening (tonic)

Involve sudden tone loss, causing slumping / collapse (atonic)

Be severe (grand mal) tonic to clonic phase, with subsequent unconsciousness, possible cyanosis, incontinence, confusion, and drowsiness on regaining consciousness

Involve sudden, brief altered consciousness (absence seizures / petit mal)

Involve a stop in motor activity, and then immediate recovery without confusion / any awareness of attack

Partial seizures possibly:

Simple or complex

Complex often arise in the temporal lobe (temporal lobe epilepsy)

Consciousness altered

Unilateral muscle-jerking

Speech affected

Sensory hallucinations, e.g. smell, taste, flashing lights, hearing

Memory / perception disorders, e.g.

     (i)   *déjà-vu*

     (ii) objects appear large or small

     (iii) feelings of unreality

Dream state

Strong emotional feelings, e.g. rage, fear, pleasure, displeasure

Confusion and automated, repetitive behaviour, e.g. chewing, gesturing, walking in circles

Management

Depends on type and frequency of seizures

Common drugs used – carbamazepine (Tegretol), phenobarbitone, phenytoin (Epanutin), sodium valporate (Epilim)

Status epilepticus = repeated major seizures without return to consciousness

Student activity:

Additional information http://www.epilepsy.com/
http://www.epilepsyfoundation.org/

Epilepsy and pregnancy

Increased congenital abnormalities (if treated / not) (screening offered), e.g.

Congenital heart (phenytoin)

Cleft lip / palate (phenobarbitone)
NTD (carbamazepine, phenytoin, valporate)

Maternal / neonatal coagulation defects (phenobarbitone)
IM vitamin K to mother during pregnancy / labour or if any bleeding
IM vitamin K to neonate

Pre-conception:
Neurological specialist advice *re* medication control
Folic acid supplements – 5 mg daily
Inform mother of potential risks

During pregnancy / postnatal:
Dangers of not treating outweigh treatment as seizures may:
  (i)   increase / decrease / not change
  (ii) re-occur after years without episodes
  (iii) present for the first time
  (iv) return to pre-pregnant state postnatally
Breastfeeding suitable with most medications
Risk of maternal death – 13 during 2000–2002 (Lewis 2004)

Student activity:
Compare / contrast epileptic seizures and eclampsia
Note your local policy for managing status epilepticus

Episiotomy (see also **perineal repair** below)
Part of the midwife's role after perineal infiltration with local anaesthetic –
  mediolateral episiotomy in UK avoiding trauma to Bartholin's glands / anal
  sphincter

Aim:
Enlarge vaginal introitus, facilitating safe delivery for mother / baby

Preparation:
Procedure carefully explained prior to labour / discuss likelihood during
  labour
Seek informed consent (NMC 2004a)
Trolley with needles, syringes, local anaesthetic (lignocaine 0.5% 10 ml or 1%
  5 ml)
Episiotomy scissors
Maintain woman's dignity

Action:
Anaesthetic:
Local anaesthetic drawn up into syringe

Woman in semi-recumbent position – perineum swabbed / antiseptic solution

Two fingers inserted into vagina; perineum lifted off fetal head

Needle inserted beneath skin, 4–5 cm along line proposed for incision

Piston of syringe withdrawn to ensure no blood

Lignocaine injected as needle slowly withdrawn, about ⅓ syringe contents

Redirect needle before fully withdrawn; make two further injections either side of original line. Fan-shaped area infiltrated – NB infiltration timing important to allow anaesthesia (unnecessary infiltration better than performing episiotomy without).

Incision:
Ideally performed during a contraction when perineum thin / distended

Place two fingers into the vagina – to protect fetal head

Open scissors, place blades along the line of infiltration

Incision made during a contraction – a single deliberate cut the length of the blades

Scissors removed / replaced on trolley

Delivery of head follows almost immediately with next contraction – be prepared

Continue as normal delivery

NB PPH possible from episiotomy; check blood loss.

Erb's palsy (paralysis)
Arm weakness / paralysis in neonate due to damaged brachial plexus (nerve group in the lower neck)

Signs:
Arm hangs loosely / palm turned backwards

Aetiology:
Neck-stretching during breech / difficult delivery

Management:
Information / explanation to parents

Physiotherapy aids resolution

Exchange transfusion

Aims:

Removal unconjugated bilirubin, antibodies and damaged cells

Correct anaemia

Prior procedures if baby at risk:

Paediatrician at birth

Immediately cord clamping / cutting – 5 cm stump left

Cord blood – group, Hb, bilirubin, Coombs test (see Section 1)

Hb < 12 g / dl / cord bilirubin > 85 μmol / l (normal 5–16 μmol / l) – immediate exchange

Hb > 14 g / dl / bilirubin < 50 μmol / dl treat as physiological jaundice

Hb < 14 g / dl / bilirubin < 50 μmol / dl exchange 4–6 hours

Preparation:

Baby in NNICU

Parents informed / supported

Blood glucose, potassium, calcium – before and during

Hb, bilirubin, blood gases, U & E before

Maintain thermal environment

Ensure clock with second-hand available

Resuscitation / monitoring equipment

? Vitamin K prior

Quieten baby – ? dummy (sedatives may mask shock)

Equipment:

      (i)   umbilical catheter

      (ii) extension tube and 3-way tap

      (ii) container for waste blood

      (iv) calcium gluconate

      (v) infusion stand and blood warmer

      (vi) record chart

Action:

Senior paediatrician / sterile procedure approx. 2 hours

Assisting midwife / nurse

Fresh Rhesus-negative, ABO-compatible blood exchanged; 170–180 ml/kg (3 kg baby = 540 ml); calcium gluconate if stored blood; counteracts citrate (anticoagulant).

Procedure ? repeated 2–3 times

Immobilise baby in splint

Stomach empty – ? give dummy

Umbilical vein technique:
Umbilical vein catheter passed – blood withdrawal / donation using 3-way tap
5–20 ml blood withdrawn and discarded
Tap turned, then equal amount donor blood replaced ? blood warmer used

Two-site technique:
Peripheral artery / umbilical artery for withdrawal
Peripheral vein for donation
5–20 ml blood withdrawn and discarded – simultaneous replacement with equal amount donor blood via Syringe pump / blood warmer
Observations:
      (i)   strict fluid balance / exchange
      (ii) vital signs – ? continuous ECG
      (iii) ? pulse oximetry
      (iv) general condition – colour, muscle tone

Post-transfusion care:
Umbilical vein / artery sutured or ligated prn
Continue observations
? Phototherapy
Repeat blood tests
Baby not fed for 2–3 hours
Parental information / support / care participation
? Oral iron later
Paediatric follow-up

Dangers:
Over-transfusion
Shock
Necrotising enterocolitis (inflamed / ischaemic / obstructed bowel)

Face presentation (see also occipito-posterior (OP) position below)
Head presenting fully flexed, occiput against shoulders

Aetiology:
Primary – i.e. before labour, due to:
Abnormal fetus, e.g. anencephalic; fetal goitre (enlarged thyroid)

Secondary – i.e. develops during labour, owing to:
Extended brow presentation
Oblique uterine position

Lax uterine muscles
Flat / abnormal pelvis
Prematurity
Polyhydramnios
Multiple pregnancy

Diagnosis:

Abdominal palpation – difficult, possibly high presenting part
VE (NB avoid trauma from examination) (see Figure 2.1)

(i)   ? high presenting part
(ii) orbital ridges / mouth felt (? sucked finger)
(iii) differentiate from anus of breech
(iv) oedema and bruising, ? identification landmarks difficult

Management – pregnancy:

USS excludes abnormalities and multiple pregnancy
? X-ray pelvimetry excludes CPD

Management – labour:

Usual care

Management – delivery (see **delivery technique** in Section 2 above)

Fainting

Sudden loss of consciousness, full / partial

Aetiology:

Not uncommon antenatally
General / supine hypotension
Anaemia
Shock – physiological / emotional

Prevention:

Avoid prolonged standing, supine position, sudden position changes, e.g. rapid
rising from bed, very warm conditions (peripheral dilatation)

Management:

Recovery position
Ensure clear airway
Medical aid / ambulance if no rapid recovery / complications
History to elicit possible cause
Advice on prevention

Fetal distress (see also **birth asphyxia** in Section 2 above)
A compromised fetus due to acute / chronic lack of O_2 (hypoxia)

Aetiology:
  Inadequate uterine circulation
  Placental insufficiency
  Cord occlusion
  Low maternal O_2
  APH
  Postmaturity
  Congenital abnormality
  Intrauterine infection
  Rhesus incompatibility
  Maternal shock – injury, haemorrhage due to:
      (i)   placental abruption
      (ii) eclampsia
      (iii) prolonged / precipitate labour
  Malpresentation, e.g. breech
  Cord compression – knot / prolapse
  Excessive sedation / analgesia
  Hypertonic uterine action
  Operative / instrumental delivery
  Shoulder dystocia

Associated factors:
Sociological:
  Low income, education
  Poor nutrition / general health
  Smoking / substance abuse
  Maternal age – >35, young teenagers

Maternal disease:
  Hypertensive disorders (chronic or pregnancy-related)
  Cardiac, chronic renal, pulmonary
  Diabetes – poorly controlled
  Severe anaemia, haemoglobinopathies
  Epilepsy – poorly controlled

Signs – chronic:
  Diminished fetal movements (FM)
  IUGR – noted on abdominal palpation

USS / Doppler USS – diminished umbilical artery / uterine vessel flow
Biophysical profile – diminished FM and breathing movements, oligohydramnios

Signs – acute and chronic:

Fetal heart auscultation – abnormalities in rate / regularity
CTG

> (i) reduced baseline variability
> (ii) non-reactive pattern, i.e. no FH accelerations
> (iii) severe bradycardia / tachycardia or reduced variability
> (iv) late decelerations
> (v) marked variable decelerations
> (vi) sinusoidal pattern

Meconium liquor
Fetal blood sample – pH at / below 7.20 (7.25 borderline)

Management – chronic:

Antenatal:

Obstetric-led care
? Manage underlying cause
Avoid strenuous exercise / work
Regular monitoring of fetal well-being
? Pre-term delivery

Labour:

Hospital birth
Obstetric-led care
Continuous CTG
? Instrumental / operative delivery
Paediatrician at delivery
? NNICU on standby

Management – acute

Medical aid – obstetric SHO / registrar
Assess labour stage
? Fetal blood sampling
? Instrumental / operative delivery
Paediatrician / midwife / nurse skilled in advanced resuscitation at delivery
  (see **birth asphyxia** in Section 2 above (resuscitation))
? NNICU on standby

Complications:
   Intrauterine death (IUD)
   Perinatal / neonatal death
   Long-term morbidity:
         (i)   poor physical / intellectual development
         (ii) cerebral palsy
   Parental and family stress / anxiety – long-term psycho-social consequences

Student activity:
Familiarise yourself with normal / abnormal CTGs
Note your local policy on calling medical aid in fetal distress
Observe biophysical profiles
Further reading: Dimond 1997; Mitchell 1995

Fitting – see **epilepsy**; **eclampsia**; **jittery (twitching) baby** in Section 2

Forceps delivery – see **instrumental delivery** in Section 2

Frequency of micturition
Abnormal frequency in PU

Aetiology:
   Physiology of pregnancy, i.e. pressure from gravid uterus on bladder
   UTI – e.g. cystitis, pyelonephritis

Management:
   History aids diagnosis
   Dip stick urinalysis
   MSSU for culture / sensitivity (C & S)

Fundal height estimation (antenatal)
Recommended by NICE 2003 (but not an exact science)

Aim:
   Locate the uterine fundus measuring distance to symphysis pubis
   Compare with previous recordings to estimate fetal growth

Preparation:
   Ensure privacy
   Woman to empty bladder
   Woman lying as flat as is comfortable (avoid supine hypotension)

Explain procedure / gain consent

Tape measure available

Wash hands

Action:

Standing on woman's right, using left hand palpate upper abdomen until fundus located – place ulnar border of hand here

Place free end of tape on upper border of symphysis pubis – extend to left hand

Note measurement in centimetres

Advise woman of findings, e.g. 30 cm = 30 weeks gestation

Record in notes / chart on growth curve

Deviation from normal – inform doctor

Fundal height estimation (postnatal)

Controversial (Cluett *et al.* 1995) – ? discontinued

Tape measuring imprecise / unhelpful when making clinical judgements

Uterine consistency / loss *per vaginam* more appropriate

Student activity:

Further reading: Cluett *et al.* 1995, NICE 2003

Haemoglobinopathies

A group of hereditary globin (protein of haemoglobin) abnormalities

Haemoglobin (Hb) – normal:

Has 4 iron (haem) atoms and 4 protein (globin) chains – half genetically from each parent

98% adult Hb = 2 alpha and 2 beta chains (HbA)

2% adult Hb = 2 alpha and 2 delta chains (HbA$_2$)

Fetal Hb = 2 alpha and 2 gamma chains – (adult Hb by 6 months)

Alpha chains = 141 amino acids (proteins or polypeptides) – each chain has 2 genes

Beta, delta and gamma chains = 146 amino acids – each chain has 1 gene

General consequences of abnormal Hb:

Changes in O_2 affinity – cyanosis and polycythaemia (excess red cells)

Unstable molecules – excess haemolysis (breakdown) rbc – anaemia

Types of haemoglobinopathies:

>300 – only 2 important in pregnancy

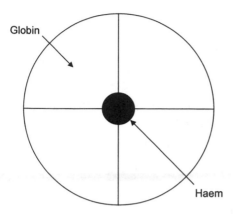

Normal haemoglobin:

Diagram 3.1 Composition

4 iron (haem) atoms and 4 protein (globin) chains

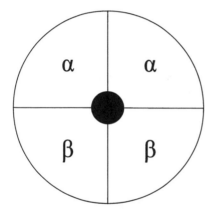

Diagram 3.2.1 HbA = 98% of adults

2 alpha and 2 beta protein chains

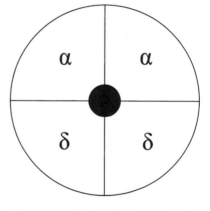

Diagram 3.2.2 HbA$_2$ = 2% of adults

2 alpha and 2 delta protein chains

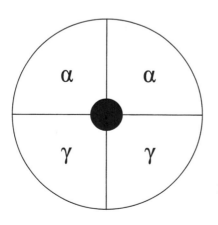

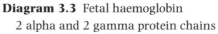

Diagram 3.3 Fetal haemoglobin

2 alpha and 2 gamma protein chains

Sickle cell disease (or sickle cell anaemia)

Mainly West Africans, West Indians – less often Indians, Greeks, Cypriots

Beta chain is affected – labelled HbS or HbC, depending on abnormality

Inherited from both parents = HbSS or HbCC or HbSC (homozygous)

Inherited from one parent = HbAS or HbAC (heterozygous) – sickle cell trait

Sickle crisis may occur (see below)

Consequences of HbSS or HbSC (HbCC no sickling occurs)

Rbc only last 17 days (normally 120)

Anaemia / possibly jaundice from excess haemolysis

Rbc sickle – (sickle cell crisis if severe) leads to:

    (i)   blocked vessels,

    (ii) soft-tissue inflammation, e.g. abdomen, lungs, joints, organs (esp. kidneys)

    (iii) hepatosplenomegaly (enlarged liver and spleen)

    (iv) stroke / death

Causes of sickle crisis

    (i)   sudden temperature change

    (ii) dehydration

    (iii) infection

    (iv) alcohol

    (v) emotional stress

Abnormal haemoglobin:

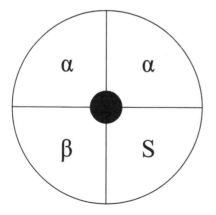

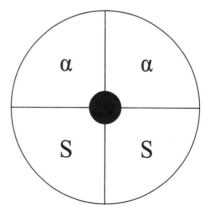

Diagram 3.4.1 Sickle cell trait
2 alpha protein chains, 1 beta protein chain, 1 sickle protein chain

Diagram 3.4.2 Sickle cell disease
2 alpha protein chains, 2 sickle protein chains

Management of a crisis

    (i) analgesia; hospitalisation if severe; hydration; prophylactic antibiotics;

    (ii) ? O_2; heparin; blood transfusion / exchange transfusion

Management in pregnancy:

Early booking (see website below *re* national screening policies)

Genetic counselling for couple (ideally pre-conception)

Diagnose fetus – CVS; amniocentesis; fetal blood via fetoscopy

Offer TOP if fetus affected

Obstetric / haematologist care

FBC, Hb

Routine infection screening, e.g. MSSU

? Prophylactic antibiotics, especially in labour

Monitor fetal growth / well-being

Liver function tests

? Blood or exchange transfusion if Hb low

Adequate hydration in labour

? O_2 especially if drowsy

No IUCD postnatally (infection risk), or combined oral contraception – progesterone-only and barrier methods suitable

Thalassaemia

World-wide, most common haemoglobinopathy – prevalent around Mediterranean area

1. Alpha thalassaemia – 6 forms – commoner in Asians / East Asians (China, Hong Kong, Singapore, Malaysia)
2. Beta thalassaemia – 10 forms – commoner in Greeks, Cypriots, Italians
3. Gamma thalassaemia – affecting fetal haemoglobin

Consequences of thalassaemia

Depends on type

Rbc last about 40 days (normal = 120) depending on severity of haemolysis

    (1) Alpha thalassaemia

        (i) alpha thalassaemia minor or trait (heterozygous) = 1–2 genes affected – asymptomatic

        (ii) 3 genes affected = very unstable – poor outcome

        (iii) alpha thalassaemia major (homozygous) = all 4 genes affected, i.e. 2 in each chain – IUD or perinatal death (therefore no adults)

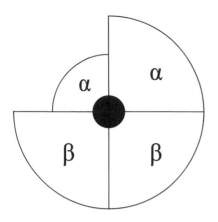

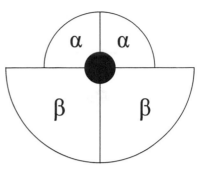

Diagram 3.5.2 Alpha thalassaemia major

Both alpha protein chains affected (i.e. all 4 genes)

Diagram 3.5.1 Alpha thalassaemia minor or trait

1 alpha protein chain affected (i.e. 1 or 2 genes)

(2) Beta thalassaemia: presents about 6 months after birth as adult Hb produced

    (i)   beta thalassaemia minor (heterozygous) = gene in 1 chain affected
- Hb often low (10 g)
- usually well
- folic acid supplement – no iron unless deficient

    (ii)   beta thalassaemia major (homozygous) = each gene in both chains affected
- hepatosplenomegaly (enlarged liver and spleen)
- bone deformities
- hypoxia and iron overload (due to haemolysis) – liver damage / heart failure
- endocrine failure – growth retardation and gonad failure = infertility
- may survive until mid-adulthood if well managed

Management in pregnancy (thalassaemia minor)

Early booking (see website below *re* national screening policies)

Genetic counselling for couple (ideally pre-conception)

Diagnose fetus – CVS; amniocentesis; fetal blood via fetoscopy

Offer TOP if fetus affected

Obstetric and haematological care

FBC and Hb

Folic acid only, unless iron-deficient

Infection screening

    (3) Gamma thalassaemia – IUD or perinatal death

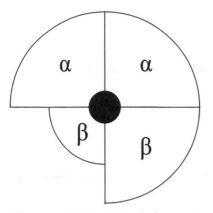

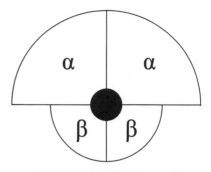

Diagram 3.6.1 Beta thalassaemia minor
  1 beta chain affected (i.e. the 1 gene)

Diagram 3.6.2 Beta thalassaemia major
  Both beta chains affected (i.e. both genes)

Student activity:

Diagramatically depict inheritance as in PKU (see **phenylketonuria (PKU)** below), but substituting HbAA, HbAS, HbSS, HbSC

Note your local policies regarding routine antenatal screening for haemoglobinopathies

Further reading:

National screening policy on http://www.kcl-phs.org.uk/haemscreening/newborn.htm

http://www.sickle-thalassaemia.org/Haemoglobin.htm

Haemorrhagic disease (Vitamin K deficient bleeding – VKDB)

Uncommon, potentially life-threatening bleeding due to lack of vitamin K 1–7 days after birth (commonly 3–4th day) or later

Aetiology:

Liver unable to synthesise clotting factors II (prothrombin); VII; IX; X owing to lack of vitamin K

Contributory factors:

Prematurity

Breastfeeding (human milk is low in vitamin K)

Slow colonisation of normal gut flora (needed for vitamin K synthesis), e.g. due to delayed or prolonged feeding or antibiotics

Perinatal hypoxia, birth asphyxia, trauma
Oral anticoagulants antenatally
Maternal anticonvulsants for epilepsy, e.g. phenobarbitone, phenytoin
Neonatal liver disease (late-onset bleeding)

Signs:

Lethargic
Pale
Irritable
Abnormal coagulation studies
Abnormal bleeding:

      (i)   from nose, mouth
      (ii)   haematemesis (vomiting blood)
      (iii) melaena (blood in faeces)
      (iv) from skin and mucous membrane
      (v)   after heel prick
      (vi) large cephalhaematoma
      (vii) brain – seen on scan

Prevention:

Avoid oral anticoagulants antenatally
Alternative anticonvulsants
Prevent prematurity / perinatal compromise
Establish early feeding
Avoid prolonged antibiotics
Routine prophylactic vitamin K (see DoH 1998) with parental consent
NB controversy *re* administration route i.e. oral / IM

Management:

Depends on severity
Blood for coagulation studies; FBC; Hb; group and cross-match
Special / intensive care
Administration / repeat vitamin K
Fresh frozen plasma
Blood transfusion
Information / support for parents

Complications:

Anaemia
Neurological damage from cerebral haemorrhage
Death

Student activity:
Note your local policy on vitamin K administration
Further reading: Karpatkin 1999; Ruby 1997, 1998

Haemorrhoids
Varicose veins in the rectum or anal area
Aetiology:
   Pre-existing prior to pregnancy /childbirth
   Chronic condition due to childbearing
   Pressure from the gravid uterus
   Progesterone relaxing smooth muscle of veins
   Straining during second-stage labour
   Obesity
   Constipation

Management:
   Avoid forced pushing during second stage
   Prevent constipation: high-fibre diet, mild laxatives, e.g. lactulose
   Topical cream / ointment prn, e.g. Anusol
   Pelvic floor exercises
   Medical aid if severe

Student activity:
Further reading: Turner 1999a

Headaches
Aetiology:
   Not uncommon antenatally / postnatally
   Stress / fatigue
   Hypertension, especially fulminating pre-eclampsia
   Drug-induced, e.g. labetalol (hypotensive)
   Epidural anaesthetic – controversial if uncomplicated – known in dural
     puncture
   Severe pyrexia

Signs and symptoms:
   Severe headache, ? associated visual disturbance, e.g. 'flashing lights'
   Headache – postural (not lying down); after dural puncture

Management:
   History aids diagnosis
   Record BP

Medical aid prn

Specific management for cause

Heartburn (see also epigastric pain in Section 2 above)

Painful, burning sensation behind sternum, +/− simultaneous acid in the throat

Aetiology:

Gastric acid reflux due to cardiac sphincter (oesophagus / stomach junction) relaxation (progesterone relaxes smooth muscle) – oesophagitis may develop

Increased abdominal pressure from gravid uterus

Specific food / drink

Management:

Advise small frequent meals, note 'trigger' foods

Avoid very fatty, spicy, acid meals

Drink between, instead of with, meals

Avoid smoking / alcohol

Avoid drinking at bedtime

Lay propped-up in bed

Antacids

? Complementary therapies

Medical aid if simple remedies fail

NB differential diagnosis of epigastric pain – see **pregnancy-induced hypertension (PIH) and pre-eclampsia; and eclampsia** in Section 2

Student activity:

Further reading: Jones 1999

Heel prick – peripheral blood sampling

Aim – sampling:

Early detection / management of:

(i) PKU / hypothyroidism – screening policy in UK at 8–10 days

(ii) haemoglobinopathies (see website below)

(iii) hypoglycaemia (blood glucose estimation), e.g. at birth, 2, 6, 12 hours prn

(iv) other tests, e.g. SBR, Hb, blood glucose

Aim – procedure:

Obtain peripheral blood for testing

Prevent undue trauma to baby's heel (see diagram of foot)

Keep accurate records

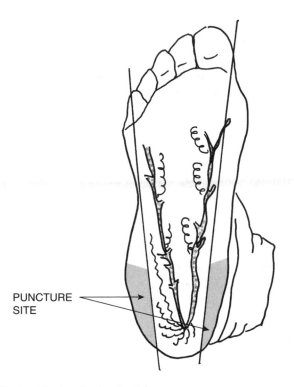

PUNCTURE
SITE

Diagram 4 Foot with sites for heel prick

Preparation:

Mother informed / consent obtained – may find it upsetting if baby cries

Check baby's identity

Accurate completion of appropriate forms

Baby comfortable / warm – especially heels

Lancet, Steret, cotton wool, plaster

Gloves worn (prevention HIV / hepatitis B transmission)

Baby held securely / lies in cot

Action:

Access heel

Massage area of foot – encourages blood flow

Swab heel – Steret

Lancet pierces skin, obtaining large blood drop

For PKU:

    (i) place drop in circle of card – ensure soaked through

    (ii) repeat until four circles filled

If capillary tube used (for other tests):

> (i) ensure adequate blood in tube and tilt to mix

For blood glucose:

> (ii) testing equipment for neonates, e.g. HemoCue™ system (more accurate for low levels than reagent strip and meter)
>
> (iii) blood squeezed on to special device
>
> (iv) placed into the machine / read at appropriate time
>
> (v) levels < 2.2 mmol / l considered significant (controversial) – ? lower without producing any signs

Apply pressure with cotton wool to stop bleeding

Plaster over puncture site

Comfort baby / give to mother

Document in records / advise mother *re* results

Appropriately record results

Student activity:

Read your unit guidelines for screening babies at risk

Further reading: Naughten 2005

National screening policy on http://www.kcl-phs.org.uk/haemscreening/newborn.htm

High vaginal swab (HVS) / speculum examination

An intimate procedure – ? causing discomfort

? Midwife's / doctor's role

HVS commonly taken when persistent / offensive vaginal discharge – using a speculum avoids contamination from the vulva / lower vagina

Cusco's speculum commonly used – after insertion two blades opened, separating vaginal walls

Speculum examination necessary to view the cervix:

> (i) in vaginal bleeding
>
> (ii) for diagnostic techniques, e.g. fibronectin detection, indicating premature labour
>
> (iii) for cervical screening

Aim:

Insert a speculum with minimum discomfort

View the cervix / upper vagina

Take HVS for detection of organisms

Use other diagnostic swabs prn

Preparation:

Explain procedure / gain consent

Dressing trolley with:

    (i)   sterile speculum, gauze swabs, sanitary towel

    (ii) disposable gloves, cleansing fluid, ? obstetric cream / lubricant (? contaminates)

    (iii) swabs / culture medium prn

Good light source

Ensure privacy

Ask woman to empty bladder

Woman placed in dorsal position, knees flexed, thighs abducted

Action:

Wash hands / apply disposable gloves

Vulva swabbed

Speculum ? lubricated / gently inserted into vagina in upward / backward direction

Open blades enabling viewing vagina / cervix

Insert swab / sweep round upper vagina / cervix to obtain specimen

Transfer to appropriate container / culture medium

Remove speculum carefully to avoid pinching vaginal walls

Dry vulva / position sanitary pad prn

Make woman comfortable

Explain result availability

Maintain accurate records

History taking

Full details:

   medical

   social

   obstetric

   present pregnancy

History taken prior to:

   'booking' a hospital bed for birth / midwife for home birth

Points to consider:

    (i)   ? 'nerve racking' experience – particularly alone / in unfamiliar surroundings – may be better to book at home

    (ii) women carry their own notes (national policy – *Changing Childbirth*: DoH 1993)

    (iii) explanation of terminology used / reasons questions asked aids understanding

    (iv) adhere to request that confidential information, e.g. TOP, not written in notes

    (v)   mothers may have difficulty remembering when faced with a barrage of questions

    (vi) history taking is more than form filling.

Aim:

Identify risk factors by taking accurate history

Form the foundations of a trusting relationship

Offer advice / information prn

Facilitate two-way discussion regarding care plans

Preparation:

Introduce yourself / other people present.

Ask what name woman / partner prefer to be called.

Put woman / partner at ease – explain procedure.

Work through history sheet – explain prn.

Use open-ended questions, e.g. ' How are you feeling?' rather than 'Do you have morning sickness?'

Write clearly / legibly – check accuracy of recorded responses.

Give discussion time, particularly over issues of family history, e.g. genetic disease / familial problems.

Discuss whether referral to other agencies required.

Provide appropriate leaflets, e.g. on healthy eating, alcohol and smoking risks (oral information may be forgotten).

? Informally discuss preliminary care plans.

Discuss other things that may arise.

Give forms / information regarding blood tests, following physical examination.

Ensure relevant telephone numbers documented.

Student activity:

Familiarise yourself with your unit's history sheet / computer systems.

List routine blood tests at the first visit.

HOOP (Hands On Or Poised) **Study**

A randomised controlled trial conducted December 1994–6 comparing perineal pain 10 days after two methods of conducting a normal delivery:

Method 1   Midwife's hands put pressure and flexion on the baby's head, i.e. to guard the perineum, with use of lateral flexion to deliver the shoulders.

Method 2   Midwife's hands were poised and prepared to prevent rapid expulsion of the head, but otherwise did not touch the perineum or shoulders.

Results:

Women felt significantly less pain with Method 1, although the episiotomy rate was lower in Method 2.

Student activity:

Further reading: McCandlish 1999; McCandlish *et al.* 1998

Hyperemesis gravidarum – see nausea and vomiting in Section 2 below

Hypoglycaemia – neonatal – see also heel prick in Section 2 above
Definition

Levels < 2.2 mmol / l considered significant (controversial) – ? lower without producing any signs

Aetiology

Commoner after birth than at any other time of life, e.g. due to:

    (i)   Birth asphyxia

    (ii)   Prematurity

    (iii)   Starvation – see **intrauterine growth retardation (IUGR)** below

    (iv)   Sepsis – see **infection – maternal; infection – neonatal** in Section 2 below

    (v)   Hypothermia

    (vi)   Transient hyperinsulinaemia – see hypoglycaemia (neonatal) under **diabetes** mellitus in Section 2 above

    (vii)   Maternal IVI dextrose in labour

    (viii)   Rhesus incompatibility

    (ix)   Congenital heart disease

    (x)   Inborn errors of metabolism:

    (xi)   glycogen storage disease

    (xii)   glucose-6-phosphatase deficiency

    (xiii)   galactosaemia

Management

Medical aid – paediatrician

NNICU if severe

Treat underlying cause if possible, e.g. infection
Early oral feeding if well enough

Hypothermia – neonatal

Thermoregulation:

Heat loss due to:
  (i) large surface area relative to body weight
  (ii) large head relative to body
  (iii) inability to shiver (muscle activity creates heat)
  (iv) conduction – direct contact
  (v) convection – air-cooled
  (vi) radiation – heat given off
  (vii) evaporation – drying moisture

Heat maintenance aided by:
  (i) drying baby
  (ii) warm room / overhead heater / incubator
  (iii) mother–infant body contact
  (iv) wrapping in warmed bedding
  (v) metabolism of brown fat* by noradrenaline (released after cold stimulates skin nerve endings)
* around kidneys, at back of neck, between shoulder blades

Risk factors:

Pre-term
  (i) little / no brown / subcutaneous fat
  (ii) immature thermoregulation centre
  (iii) low glycogen stores

Small for gestational age
  (i) little / no brown / subcutaneous fat
  (ii) low glycogen stores

Birth asphyxia / prolonged resuscitation – acidosis; cold O_2; exposure
Open lesions, e.g. exomphalus, spina bifida – heat loss
Hypoglycaemia – reduced energy for metabolism
Respiratory distress – altered metabolism / temperature control
Sepsis – altered metabolism / temperature control
Cerebral haemorrhage – shock; altered metabolism / temperature control

Complications:
Metabolic acidosis
Respiratory distress / RDS

Apnoea
Hypoglycaemia
Death

Identification of newborn at birth

Aim:
Accurately identify the newborn
Ensure baby is given to correct parent(s)
Parent(s) / witness(es) identification

Preparation:
Two identity bands with:
(i) maternal surname, maternal / baby case note number
(ii) infant's first name, date / time of birth.
Ask mother / partner to check details whilst in labour ward.

Action:
Promptly after birth, securely attach to baby's ankle(s) / wrist in presence of
parent(s); ensure bands not too tight / loose.
Document details in case records.
? Write cot card with same information plus sex / weight.
Two midwives check bands if an unaccompanied woman has had a GA.
On receiving to ward identity bands checked / records signed.
If one band becomes detached midwife informed; details checked again with
mother; new band applied.
If both bands detached – two midwives check all babies before reapplying iden-
tity bands to the unnamed baby.

Student activity:
Identify your local protocol

Incontinence

Involuntary passage of urine / faeces
Frequent, intermittent, during stress, e.g. coughing, sneezing, laughing – ?
retention with overflow

Aetiology:
Pressure from gravid uterus
UTI
Bladder damage, especially to bladder neck, during labour / delivery
Pelvic floor damage (nerves, muscle, connective tissue)

Poor muscle tone, including anal sphincter

Fistulae between vagina and bladder (vesico-vaginal) or vagina and rectum (recto-vaginal)

Management:

Prevention / early treatment of UTI

Ensure bladder emptied after PU

Prevent constipation

Avoid pelvic floor trauma, e.g. instrumental delivery / prolonged second stage.

Early trauma detection / treatment

Indwelling urinary catheter if severe trauma

Pelvic floor exercises

Induction of labour – alternative and 'natural'

Alternative methods of increasing circulating oxytocin / prostaglandins – possibly useful if there is no urgency

Methods:

Membrane sweeping:

vaginal examination is performed, finger enters cervix to sweep the lower uterine segment to detach the membranes – may cause woman considerable discomfort, some bleeding and irregular contractions

(In strict privacy, usually only at home!)

Nipple stimulation

Clitoral stimulation

Sexual intercourse (prostaglandins are high in seminal fluid)

Student activity:

Further reading: Boulvain *et al.* 2005

Induction of labour – medical

(see also **augmentation / acceleration of labour** in Section 2 above)

? Midwife's role in uncomplicated cases following medical discussion (see Rule 6 in *Midwives' Rules and Standards*: NMC 2004b)

Indications:

Postmaturity

Hypertensive disorders

Medical conditions – renal / heart disease, diabetes

PROM

Placental abruption (not requiring emergency caesarean section)

Previous obstetric history, e.g. stillbirth

Unstable lie (once corrected) (see **transverse / oblique lie** in Section 2 below)

Fetal compromise – IUGR; rhesus isoimmunization

IUD

Severe congenital abnormality

Maternal request (controversial)

Contraindications:

Maternal objection

Major CPD

Transverse / oblique lie

Severe fetal compromise

Placenta praevia

Severe APH

Cautious use:

Minor CPD

Multigravidas

IUGR

Compromised fetus

Uterine scar

Methods:

Depends on gestation / indication

1 *Prostaglandin* – used for:

  (i)   cervical ripening / softening
  (ii) pre-term pregnancy (more successful than Syntocinon)
  (iii) IUD

Procedure:

  administration ? midwife's role in uncomplicated cases

  oral tablets / IVI solutions rarely used

  commonly vaginal gel / tablets into posterior fornix, e.g.:

  (i)   Prostin E_2 (PGE_2)
  (ii) Propess (slow release prostin – expensive)

Produces:

  local cervical action / systemic uterine action

  individual sensitivity:

  (i)   ? rapid onset of strong painful contractions
  (ii) ? very rapid labour progression

2 *ARM* (forewater amniotomy) (see also **augmentation / acceleration of labour** in Section 2 above)

3 *Syntocinon IV infusion* (see also **augmentation / acceleration of labour** in Section 2 above)

Student activity:
Note your local policy and procedures
Familiarise yourself with labour records
Revise physiology of labour
Further reading: NICE 2001b

Infection – maternal
Location:
    Upper / lower genital tract
    Systemic, i.e. general
    Urinary tract
    Breast
    Coexisting, e.g. tonsillitis, appendicitis

Pre-disposing factors:
    Social disadvantage
    Poor nutrition, poor hygiene
    Poor general health; medical conditions, e.g. anaemia, diabetes
    Exposure to infection, e.g. STIs, contaminated food, cross-infection
    Stress / anxiety
    Prolonged / difficult labour
    Surgical procedures / trauma
    Retained products of conception

Types of organisms:
    Bacteria
    Viruses
    Fungi
    Protozoa
    Spirochetes
    Parasites

Prevention:
    Improve nutrition / hygiene, especially hand-washing
    Safe sexual practice (pregnancy = unprotected intercourse)
    Early identification / management of infection, especially UTI / genital tract

Ensure bladder emptied when PU
Correct anaemia
Avoid exposure to infections
Effective labour management
Prevent prolonged labour /dehydration
Aseptic technique
Minimal intervention, e.g. VEs / catheterisation
Minimise trauma
Prophylactic antibiotics in 'risk' cases
Avoid rough handling of breasts
Correct fixing when breastfeeding

Complications:

Intrauterine infection – miscarriage; IUD; congenital abnormalities / infection
Perinatal death
Pre-term labour / PROM
Maternal morbidity:
>   (i)   physical – renal damage, scar tissue, secondary PPH
>   (ii)   psychological – fear of future pregnancies, resentment towards partner / baby
>   (iii) psycho-sexual – loss of libido, dyspareunia (painful intercourse)
>   (iv)   social – unwilling / unable to fulfil normal social life

Maternal mortality:
13 deaths from genital tract infection between 2000 and 2002 (Lewis 2004)

Management

Depends on location of infection – early recognition and treatment essential
see Libbus 2001; Thompson in Lewis 2001, p. 121 and Harper in Lewis 2004, Chapter 7

Infection – neonatal

Infection during the first 28 days of life:
Early onset <5 days (average 20 hours)
Late onset >5 days (average 20 days)

Neonatal defences:

Intact skin
White blood cells inefficient, especially following hypothermia
Immunoglobulins:

(i)   IgG – transplacental, i.e. passive immunity (low pre-term)
(ii) IgA – low levels (synthesised from 30 weeks gestation)
(iii) IgM – low levels (present from 13 weeks gestation); increases following infection / oral feeding
(iv) IgA – from colostrum and breast milk

High-risk factors:

Maternal infection	– general; intrauterine; vaginal
Membranes	– prolonged rupture; ARM; meconium-stained; amnionitis
Monitoring labour	– FSE; vaginal examinations
Labour	– prolonged; premature; difficult
Delivery	– difficult; operative
Compromised baby	– perinatal hypoxia; asphyxia; vigorous resuscitation; meconium aspiration; prematurity (low IgG levels); IUGR; multiple pregnancy; hypothermia; congenital abnormality; admission to neonatal unit – procedures; cross-infection

Routes of infection:

Ascending vaginal flora	– anaerobic bacteria; *Streptococcus* (strep.) *pneumoniae*; *E. coli*; group B strep.
Transplacental	– rubella; *Listeria*; syphilis; gonorrhoea; *Varicella zoster* (chickenpox – a notifiable disease); HIV; toxoplasmosis
Intrapartum	– gonorrhoea; *Chlamydia*; *Herpes*; *Candida* (thrush)
Cross-infection	– *Streptococcus epidermidis*; *Staphylococcus aureus*; haemolytic strep.; some viruses
Breastfeeding	– HIV; yeasts

Signs and symptoms:
General:

Pyrexia
Hypothermia
Temperature instability
Weak cry
Pallor
Failure to thrive
Jaundice
Skin rash / pustules

Neurological:
   Lethargy
   Irritability
   High-pitched cry
   Convulsions / jittery baby
   Hypotonia/ hypertonia
   Neck rigidity
   Full fontanelle

Respiratory:
   Tachypnoea / apnoea
   Intercostal recession
   Grunting
   Changes on X-ray

Cardiovascular:
   Tachycardia / bradycardia
   Central cyanosis
   Anaemia
   Thrombocytopenia (low platelets)
   Abnormal white cell count

Gastrointestinal:
   Poor feeding
   Abdominal distension
   Vomiting
   Diarrhoea
   Blood in stool (melaena)
   Enlarged liver / spleen

Diagnosis:
   Signs and symptoms; history
   Early-onset recognition difficult
   First 24 hours only – gastric aspirate / external auditory canal (ear) swab
   Blood – culture; FBC; ESR and IgM (raised in infection)
   Culture – nose, throat, cord, rectal swabs; urine; endotracheal tube and IVI
      tips
   Lumbar puncture – culture CSF
   X-ray – chest; abdomen
   Ultrasound scan, e.g. brain

Management:

Depends on condition / severity

Medical aid (paediatrician, or GP if mild late-onset)

Complications:

General infection

Skin infections

Pyoderma (septic spots)

Pemphigus neonatorum

Candida (thrush – buttocks)

Paronychia (nail bed)

Mucous membrane – oral *Candida*

Umbilical cord (risk of systemic spread)

Septicaemia (growth of organisms in blood)

Meningitis

Pneumonia

UTI

Gastro-enteritis

Ophthalmia neonatorum (eye infection)

Necrotising enterocolitis (NEC) – inflamed necrotic bowel

Student activity:

Consider antenatal advice on prevention

Review local preventive practice during labour

Elicit protocol for obtaining medical aid in the community

Further reading: Bott 1999b; Bott 2000b; Davis 1998; Dyke 1998; Greer 1998; Nicholas 1998; Percival 2003; Smith 1998; Weston 1998a, b; Wright 1998

Initial newborn examination

Part of midwife's role following delivery – mother / father present

'Top to toe' physical examination and auscultation heart / lungs – ? paediatric role or extended role of midwife

Aim:

Detection of abnormalities

Record findings accurately in case notes

Inform mother / father of findings

Alert paediatrician prn

Preparation:
Explain procedure to parent(s) – invite observation
Maintain baby's temperature (see **hypothermia – neonatal** above in Section 2)

Action:
Assess Apgar score prior to examination
Observe muscle tone / response to stimuli
Listen to the cry / ? colour changes
Axillary temperature
Two people weigh – inform parent(s) / record
Measure length / head circumference prn
Work from head to toe:

(i) head – size, shape, symmetry of skull: feel suture lines / fontanelles

(ii) face – ? two normal eyes, which both open

(iii) nose – two patent nostrils

(iv) lips / mouth – ? cleft lip / palate, teeth, 'tongue tie'

(v) ? chin normally developed

(vi) ? ears normal shape / structure, position on head (? in line with the eyebrows)

(vii) neck – front / back ? abnormal swellings

(viii) skin folds / pads of fat between shoulders

(ix) arms – ? normal length compared to body, normal position / joints

(x) hands – count digits; check for webbing / abnormal appendages; examine palmar creases

(xi) chest – ? symmetrical; ? normal rib cage / diaphragm movement, normal nipples for gestation

(xii) abdomen – ? normal configuration / cord insertion; ? swellings / abnormalities / gut / abnormal discharges

(xiii) genitalia – boys – ? urethral opening at tip of penis, normal scrotum / descended testes; ? abnormal swellings

(xiv) genitalia – girls – ? normal labia – separate ? normal urethra / vagina openings

(xv) anus – ? normal situation / patency

(xvi) hips – test for dislocation / instability (see **Barlow's test** – Section 1) – ? paediatric role

(xvii) legs – ? normal length compared to body / appearance / position; ? normal knee joint

(xviii) feet – ? position; count digits; check for webbing / abnormal
appendages

(xix) back – run fingers along length ? abnormal indentations / swellings
/ hair tufts;

(xx) neural tube openings obvious

Document findings in records.

Student activity:
Further reading: Williamson *et al.* 2005

Insomnia
Inability to sleep

Aetiology:
Physiological / psychological

Discomfort of gravid uterus, especially in late pregnancy

Minor disorders of pregnancy – heartburn, cramp

Frequency of micturition

Anxiety / worry about pregnancy, baby, own health, sociological factors

Depression, ? early sign postnatally

Bereavement

Management:
Depends on cause

Change of position during pregnancy

Investigate frequency of micturition

Effective communication: enable the expression of concerns / anxieties

Information prn

Encourage family support / practical help

Counselling prn

Early identification / treatment depression

Instrumental delivery
Forceps delivery:

Speeds delivery of fetal head – protects fetus / mother from undue trauma /
exhaustion

Not a midwife's role

Prerequisites:
Cervix fully dilated

Bladder empty

Membranes ruptured

Head engaged
Denominator identified
Effective uterine contractions
Adequate anaesthesia
Episiotomy
Informed consent

Aims

Assist obstetrician
Support woman / partner throughout
Maintain contemporaneous records

Preparation:

Two midwives – assist obstetrician / receive baby
Trolley prepared for normal delivery
Sterile pack obstetric forceps – obstetrician determines type:
    (i)   deep rotational, e.g. Kielland's
    (ii) mid-cavity delivery, e.g. Neville Barnes's, Haig Ferguson's, Simpson's
    (iii) low-cavity delivery, e.g. Wrigley's
Adequate needles, syringes, local anaesthetic, suture materials
Inform paediatrician
Effective resuscitation equipment

Action:

Place woman in lithotomy position, wedge under one side (prevents supine
    hypotension)
Open forceps pack / required equipment, e.g. for infiltration / pudendal nerve
    block
Keep woman / partner informed of progress
Advise woman *re* pushing prn
Midwife receives baby as normal – shows to mother / passes to paediatrician
    (ID labels)
Syntometrine given with birth of anterior shoulder unless contraindicated
Assist with perineal repair
Remove legs from stirrups / make woman comfortable

Ventouse delivery (may be part of midwife's extended role)

Speeds delivery fetal head
? Prevents caesarean section in late first-stage labour

Prerequisites:

As for forceps delivery, but cervix may be present

Aims: As for forceps delivery

Preparation:

As for forceps, but substitute sterile silastic cups, tubing, vacuum extractor (electronic or hand pump), metal chain and handle

Action:

Presentation confirmed

Silastic cup applied to fetal head as near to occiput as possible

Vacuum applied slowly from $0.2\,kg/cm^2$ to $0.8\,kg/cm^2$

Ensure cup secure / apply steady downward traction as the mother pushes

Head rotated if necessary

Episiotomy prn

Use steady gentle traction to follow the arc of the curve of Carus (see Section 1) through the pelvis and continue forward and upward as the head is born, i.e. continuing the curve.

Cup removed carefully

Syntometrine given with birth of anterior shoulder unless contraindicated

Continue as for forceps delivery

After birth:

Perform initial observations

Maintain records accurately

NB – increased complication risk for mother / baby ? observe longer in labour ward

Discuss reasons for instrumental delivery with mother

Advise mother that chignon (large bruised swelling) will subside after ventouse

Student activity:

Further reading Hamilton 2003

Intrauterine death (IUD)

Fetal death. Expulsion of fetus = miscarriage at <24 weeks, or stillbirth >24 weeks

Aetiology:

Often unknown

Chronic maternal causes:

    (i)   diabetes

    (ii) cardiac, respiratory, renal disease

(iii) essential hypertension

(iv) smoking, substance abuse

(v) low socio-economic status

(vi) cholestasis

Acute maternal causes:

(i) PIH / pre-eclampsia / eclampsia

(ii) systemic infection, e.g. toxoplasmosis; viral; bacterial

(iii) STIs, e.g. syphilis; herpes

(iv) intrauterine infections, e.g. viral; bacterial

Placental causes:

(i) poor implantation

(ii) poor function – poor uterine blood flow, infarcts (small, old abruptions)

(iii) abruption

(iv) cord knot / entanglement / compression

Fetal causes:

(i) congenital abnormality, e.g. cardiac

(ii) IUGR

(iii) postmaturity

(iv) malpresentation

(v) shoulder dystocia

(vi) Rhesus incompatibility

(vii) intrauterine infection

Uterine causes:

(i) hypertonic uterine action

(ii) ruptured uterus

(iii) obstructed labour

Minimising risk:

(i) well-balanced maternal diet

(ii) folic acid supplements (pre-conception and early pregnancy)

(iii) vitamins supplements prn

(iv) stop smoking / avoid passive smoking

(v) avoid infection

(vi) avoid sudden illicit drug withdrawal

(vii) obstetric team management when 'at risk'

(viii) specialist liaison, e.g. physician prn

(ix) maternal information on recognition / rapid reporting of: (a) complications, e.g. bleeding, infection; (b) abnormal / absent fetal movements

(x) effective monitoring of maternal / fetal well-being

(xi) early / prompt intervention prn

Signs:

Absent FM

No FH auscultated with Pinard's stethoscope / sonic aid

No FH / FM on USS

X-ray:

(i) Spalding's sign (skull bones overlapping)

(ii) Robert's sign (gas in vessels / heart)

Management:

Antenatal:

Sensitive information to mother / family

Psychological support

Informed choice about options:

(i) await spontaneous abortion / labour

(ii) generally hospital birth, ? mother's wish home birth

(iii) induced abortion / labour

Blood for FBC, Hb, clotting screening – weekly until delivered

Labour – known IUD:

Senior obstetric management

Usual physical care

Provide:

(i) privacy / quiet room

(ii) continuity of care / experienced midwife

(iii) information / support to woman / family

Neonatal resuscitation equipment / CTG monitor removed from room

Cot remains

Ensure up-to-date blood results, especially clotting profile

Discuss analgesia *

Discuss choices:

(i) seeing / holding / bathing baby

(ii) naming baby

(iii) keepsake, e.g. lock of hair, hand- / footprint, photograph of baby / family (if unwanted initially kept in case note and available later)

(iv) post-mortem examination

(v) religious support / ceremony

(vi) funeral / cremation – (hospital can arrange cremation)

De-briefing / support for staff

Postnatal:

    Information ? repeated, supported with written details (see Dimond 2002
      Chapter 8)

    De-briefing counselling

    Family support**

    ? Contraception / pre-conception advice

    Follow-up obstetric / paediatric appointment – 6 weeks

    ? Support agencies referral

    GP / HV liaison

    Staff de-briefing / support

* totally pain-free / heavily sedated labour experience may leave the mother with unreal feeling – unfulfilled meaningless experience / lack of achievement, almost negating pregnancy

** inform family that leaving baby clothes / equipment ? helps the grieving process – ? prevents negation of pregnancy

Student activity:

Note your local policy and procedures

Further reading: Foster 1996

http://www.doh.gov.uk/ (SB / perinatal mortality statistics)

Intrauterine growth retardation (IUGR)

Aetiology:

Often unknown – ? maternal / fetal

Poor maternal health:

    Major organ disease – lungs, heart, kidney

    Hypertension – existing; pre-eclampsia; PIH

    Diabetes

    Blood disorders – severe anaemia; sickle cell disease

    Epilepsy (poorly controlled)

    Severe infection

    Poor nutrition – ? linked to social deprivation

    Smoking, drug, alcohol abuse

Fetal / placental conditions:

    Placental insufficiency after abruption

    Some congenital abnormalities, e.g. heart and renal

    Intrauterine infection – rubella, *Cytomegalovirus*, toxoplasmosis

    Rhesus incompatibility

Management

Early recognition

    (i)   USS for serial growth measurements

    (ii) biophysical profile, noting fetal limb / body / breathing movements and tone

    (iii) amniotic fluid levels

    (iv) doppler studies, noting umbilical artery blood flow

Treat cause if possible, e.g. hypertension, anaemia

Avoid prolonged pregnancy

Delivery in consultant unit with NNICU (if transferring, accompanied by a trained escort)

? Pre-term delivery, induction of labour / caesarean section

Careful monitoring during labour

Paediatrician at delivery

Complications:

Intrauterine death

Perinatal death

Fetal distress in labour

Birth asphyxia

Meconium aspiration

Those associated with small for gestational age (SGA) / prematurity

Intravenous infusion (IVI) – insertion / care IV cannula

Insertion IV cannula ? midwife's role – after correct training / according to unit policy

Aim:

Establish venous access for IVI

Prevent infection

Keep accurate records

Preparation:

Dressing trolley / tray for aseptic technique

Venflon, swabs, micropore tape, tourniquet, sharps box

Transparent sterile dressing

IVI fluid, giving set, pump / stand

Procedure explained / consent gained

Choose site for woman's comfort – e.g. left arm if right-handed

IVI chart

Action – insertion:

Disposable gloves worn
Apply tourniquet; check for prominent veins
Cleanse area
Open Venflon aseptically
Insert into vein
Ensure blood flow
Cover / secure with transparent sterile dressing
IVI fluid run through giving set / threaded through pump
Ensure no air in system / connect to Venflon
Record in records / IVI chart
Check infusion site regularly ? swelling, redness, tenderness

Action – removal

Disconnect infusion
Undo dressing / tape holding cannula in place
Gauze swab over insertion area
Apply pressure / remove Venflon slowly
Maintain pressure to stop bleeding / apply dressing
Discard Venflon safely
Record date / time

Jaundice
Maternal – aetiology

Severe hyperemesis gravidarum (pregnancy sickness)
Hepatitis (liver inflammation) due to infection, often viral; or drugs
Liver damage, e.g. due to severe pre-eclampsia / eclampsia; alcoholism
Cholestasis, i.e. impaired liver function (see **cholestasis** in Section 2 above)
Obstructed biliary tract

Management:

Urgent medical aid
Treat underlying cause

Neonatal – aetiology

Physiological jaundice:

(i) common, in normal baby generally uncomplicated (exacerbated / serious if pre-term)

(ii) haemolysis (breakdown) of surplus erythrocytes (liver unable to cope with increased bilirubin) possibly due to late cord clamping (especially after Syntocinon) or strong uterine contractions leading to increased blood volume

    (iii) breastfeeding – breast milk causes alteration of bilirubin metabolism.

    (iv) haematoma – haemolysis of large haematoma / bruising increases bilirubin levels

    (v) drugs – e.g. diazepam (Valium); salicylates (aspirin).

Haemolytic jaundice:

    abnormal rbc breakdown – maternal antibodies from ABO or Rhesus incompatibility

Infection:

    (i) intrauterine – rubella, toxoplasmosis, *Cytomegalovirus*

    (ii) neonatal – viruses, bacteria – UTI, cord infections, septicaemia.

Obstruction:

    congenital biliary tract abnormalities

Metabolic:

    inborn errors of metabolism / enzyme disorders, e.g.

        (a) cystic fibrosis

        (b) hypothyroidism

        (c) galactosaemia

Miscellaneous:

    increased haemolysis due to:

        (a) large intake of maternal IVI glucose / IVI oxytocin

        (b) traumatic birth

Prevention:

Avoid prematurity; birth trauma; excess IVI glucose / oxytocin; causative drugs

Prompt cord clamping in active third stage of labour

Early feeding minimises physiological jaundice

Early recognition / management of blood incompatibilities (particularly if antibodies)

Prevention of intrauterine / neonatal infections

Management:

Maternal history

    Blood group and antibodies

    Antenatal / intrapartum health

Neonatal history

    Onset / depth of jaundice (in good light)

    General condition – alertness, feeding, urine / stool colour, signs of infection

Notify paediatrician if moderate / severe; symptomatic (see activities of a midwife, *EU Second Midwifery Directive 80/155/EEC* in NMC 2004b)

Investigations

Bilicheck (see Briscoe *et al.* 2002)

Blood for SBR, FBC, Hb, group, antibodies, U & E

Infection screening – culture urine, blood, swabs, ? CSF (lumbar puncture)

Screening for metabolic disorders

Admission to NNU prn

Phototherapy / Biliwrap / Bilibed

Drugs

(i) Phenobarbitone aids bilirubin metabolism – used cautiously (sedative effect ? inhibit feeding)

(ii) Oral iron to correct anaemia (caused by rbc haemolysis)

Exchange transfusion

In severe cases of haemolytic disease, sepsis or anaemia

Parental care

Information / support, encourage breastfeeding / participation in special care

Complications:

Anaemia

Poor feeding

Consequences of underlying cause of prematurity, infection

Kernicterus (yellow staining of brain tissue)

Student activity:

Further reading: Briscoe *et al.* 2002; Percival 2003; Waters 1996

Jittery (twitching) baby

Small trembling limb movements, ? accompanying eye movements (convulsion more obvious)

Aetiology:

Cerebral irritation

(i) hypoxia

(ii) infection

(iii) jaundice

(iv) drug withdrawal

(v) metabolic disorders, e.g. hypoglycaemia, hypomagnesaemia, hypocalcaemia (low blood sugar, magnesium, calcium); hypernatraemia (high blood sodium)

Management:

Notify paediatrician (see activities of a midwife, *EU Second Midwifery Directive 80/155/EEC* in NMC 2004b)

Identify cause

    (i) history

    (ii) observation

Screening

    (i) infection

    (ii) blood – FBC; glucose, bilirubin, electrolytes, gases

Anticonvulsants, e.g. phenobarbitone

Treat cause

Information / reassure parents

Complications:

Convulsions – cerebral anoxia, brain damage, death

Ketonuria

Urine contains ketone bodies (acetone)

Aetiology:

Fat metabolism, due to lack of carbohydrate – waste product = acetone

Cause:

Lack of insulin for carbohydrate metabolism, i.e. diabetes

Inadequate carbohydrate intake, e.g. severe vomiting

Excessive carbohydrate metabolism, e.g. prolonged labour

Dehydration aggravates condition

Management:

Treat cause appropriately

Carbohydrate replacement, e.g. oral fluids / food; IVI glucose

Urinalysis

Fluid balance

Local Supervising Authority (LSA)

In accordance with the 1997 Nurses, Midwives and Health Visitors Act, health authorities (England and Wales), health boards (Scotland), and health and social services (Northern Ireland) must stand as LSAs controlling the standards of midwifery services and practitioners. All midwives (employed or independent) must have a designated supervisor of midwives (herself a practising midwife). Supervisors provide professional support and guidance; monitor individual and unit practices; have a disciplinary role in cases of alleged misconduct; and must ensure that midwives practise legally.

Student activity:
Note references to LSA in your *Midwives' Rules and Standards* (NMC 2004b).
    Identify your local supervisors; discuss their duties.

MAGPIE trial
An international, randomised trial involving more than 80 hospitals in over 23
    countries. Recruitment began in 1998, aiming to obtain 14,000 women. Coordinated in Oxford, the trial compared mortality and morbidity following IV
    treatment of pre-eclampsia. Clinical information was collected in hospital until
    postnatal discharge; at three months with a postal survey; at four years at child
    follow-up.
Further reading: Duley and Watkins 1999

Malpresentation – fetus
A presentation other than vertex (NB not malposition of the vertex)
(see **breech**; **face presentation**; and **brow presentation** in Section 2 above;
    and **transverse / oblique lie** in Section 2 below)

Aetiology – consider:
Powers:
    uterine /abdominal muscles
Passages:
        (i) uterus – shape, liquor volume, structural anomalies
        (ii) pelvic shape / size
Passenger:
        (i) fetal size / position
        (ii) placental position

Maternity Alliance
A national charity working to improve the rights of and services for pregnant
    women, new parents and their families. A pressure group, with professional
    and lay members. The organisation provides information, support and education personally, and through literature and conferences.

2–6 Northburg St	professional advice line 0845 601 3386
London EC1V 0AY	email office@maternityalliance.org.uk
	http://www.maternityalliance.org.uk

Maternity benefits

Free prescriptions in pregnancy and for 12 months post-delivery
Free dental care in pregnancy and for 12 months post-delivery
Free eye tests and chiropody in some cases
Free milk for low-income families
Paid time off for antenatal care (proof of attendance required by employer)
Paid time off for parent education if during work time

Monetary benefits could include:

Statutory maternity pay (SMP)
Maternity allowance (MA)
Incapacity benefit (ICA) – if not entitled to the others
Statutory sick pay (SSP)
Sure Start maternity grant (if on low income)
Leave entitlement could include:

      (i)   Maternity leave – ordinary and additional
      (ii) Paternity leave
      (iii) Parental leave
      (iv) Adoption leave (SAL) and Pay
      (v) Additional Maternity Leave (AML):

Student activity:

Further details on http:/www.dwp.gov.uk/

Maternity Services Liaison Committees

A multidisciplinary committee of local personnel, e.g. member of health authority; head of midwifery; obstetrician; GP; health visitor; lay person (e.g. NCT)
monitoring the quality of maternity services and health outcomes, and offering
advice on service provision.

Meconium liquor (see also **fetal distress** in Section 2 above)

Meconium-stained liquor:
   Fresh = thick, obvious stool
   Old = passed during pregnancy – prolonged dark staining

Aetiology:

Fetal hypoxia – increased gut peristalsis and relaxation of anal sphincter
Breech presentation
Postmaturity

Management:
Antenatal:

    (i)   identify cause

    (ii) monitor fetal well-being

    (iii) ? amnioinfusion with saline to dilute

    (iv) ? deliver

Labour:

    (i)   continuous CTG

    (ii) close liquor observation

    (iii) paediatrician, midwife, nurse skilled in advanced resuscitation at delivery

    (iv) airway suction under direct vision, i.e. using laryngoscope / via ET tube

Complications:

    (i)   Meconium aspiration:

        (a) *in utero* – fetal gasping movements

        (b) at birth – baby gasps, inhaling secretions in pharynx / trachea

    (ii) Birth asphyxia

    (iii) Respiratory distress / RDS

    (iv) Chemical pneumonitis (inflamed lungs)

    (v) Pneumothorax – air into chest cavity, via damaged / collapsed alveoli

    (vi) Perinatal / neonatal death

    (vii) Long-term morbidity

Mendelson's Syndrome

Damaged respiratory tract from inhaled acidic vomit causing bronchial tree / alveoli spasm; resulting in scarring, respiratory distress, cyanosis, and tachycardia

Aetiology:

Vomiting caused by:

    (i)   slow gastric emptying / lax cardiac sphincter (progesterone influence)

    (ii) gravid uterus displacing stomach

    (iii) side-effect of pethidine / anaesthetic

Prevention:

(NB critical times = induction of anaesthesia / initial recovery)

    Routine nil by mouth prior to elective surgery

? Nil by mouth during normal labour (see Baker 1996; Newton and Champion 1997; Sharp 1997)

Routine administration oral antacid during labour / prior to surgery, e.g. ranitidine (Zantac), inhibits the production of gastric acid.

IM antiemetic with initial pethidine, e.g. prochlorperazine (Stemetil), metoclopramide (Maxolon)

Vigilance during anaesthetic induction – Sellick's manoeuvre (cricoid pressure)

Experienced obstetric anaesthetist

Recovery position / careful observation post-op.

Readily available, effective suction equipment

Management:

Maintain respiratory function / blood gas levels

Special care in an ICU, mechanical ventilation prn

Prevent complications, e.g. respiratory infection

Information / support for woman, family

Complications:

Long-term morbidity from damaged respiratory tract

Mortality:

2 deaths, plus contributory factor in others during 1988–90 (Hibbard *et al.* 1994),

1 death during 1991–93 (Hibbard *et al.* 1996)

none during 1994–96 (Lewis 1998) and 1997–1999 (Lewis 2001)

Student activity:

Further reading: Berry 1997

Mid-stream specimen urine (MSSU)

Aim:

To obtain uncontaminated specimen for laboratory testing – commonly culture and sensitivity (C & S) / ward testing

Preparation:

Explain procedure

Swabs for cleansing area

Sterile container

Correctly labelled laboratory forms

Action:

Instruct woman to wash genitalia

Initial urine flow into toilet, catch mid-stream specimen into receiver / container

Finish passing urine into toilet
Appropriately labelled container / forms to laboratory prn
Ward testing:
>   (i)   observe colour, odour, ? debris
>   (ii) insert reagent strip / time according to manufacturer's instructions
>   (iii) read results

Record in notes.

Multiple pregnancy / births
Simultaneous development of two / more embryos

Incidence:
Increased due to assisted fertility treatment

Diagnosis:
Ultrasound (early pregnancy)
Abdominal palpation:
>   (i)   uterus large for dates / many fetal parts felt (suspected)
>   (ii) three poles (buttocks / head) identified
>   (iii) two fetal hearts heard with difference >10 bpm

Pregnancy:
Possibly normal

Complications:
Exaggerated minor disorders
Increased fluid retention (increased hormones)
Low-lying placenta (large placental site)
Polyhydramnios
Malpresentation
Anaemia
PIH / pre-eclampsia
UTI

Management:
Pregnancy:
Treat complications prn
Discuss with mother – vaginal delivery / caesarean section prn
Hospital birth advised – if mother's informed choice is home, notify supervisor of midwives

Labour:

First stage:

    (i)   senior obstetrician's care

    (ii) depends on maternal condition, fetal lie / presentation

    (iii) ARM / Syntocinon with great caution prn

    (iv) usual labour care

    (v) sedatives / analgesia used cautiously (? small babies); epidural appropriate

    (vi) ? continuous electronic monitoring (twin machines available)

    (vii) prepare room for two babies, e.g. delivery pack / cots / resuscitation equipment

    (viii) obstetrician, paediatrician, anaesthetist, NNU on standby

Second stage – anticipated vaginal delivery:

    (i)   obstetrician / paediatrician present – midwife delivery/ies if cephalic

    (ii) **no** Syntometrine with first delivery

    (iii) identify first twin and placental end of cord (e.g. 1 cord clamp)

    (iv) palpate abdomen to confirm lie / presentation / FH

    (v) VE to confirm presentation / position / station

    (vi) ARM if suitable / uterus contracting – ? Syntocinon if not contracting

    (vii) vaginal delivery if cephalic / breech – caesarean section if complications

    (viii) Syntometrine IM with second delivery

    (ix) identify second twin and placental end of cord (e.g. 2 cord clamps)

Third stage:

    (i)   as normal – beware of risk of PPH

    (ii) Syntocinon infusion continued for 1–2 hours

    (iii) placental examination as normal; note number of placentae as potential indicator of zygosity

Postnatal:

    (i)   physical / psychological / practical adjustment needed

    (ii) breastfeeding possible

    (iii) extra support from midwife initially prn

    (iv) family support at home prn – ? financial help / child care for higher multiples

    (v) ? support from voluntary organisations, e.g. TAMBA (see below)

Neonates:

    (i)   remain with mother if conditions allow

    (ii) NNU if necessary

National Childbirth Trust (NCT)

A national voluntary organisation based in London with local branches and
members: a pressure group campaigning to improve maternity services, with
some research being undertaken and educational activities via publications
and study days. Volunteers offer information / support in pregnancy, childbirth
and early parenthood: parent education classes (a fee usually required) and
breastfeeding support (usually by phone but occasionally hospital / home
visits). The organisation tries to make services, activities and membership fully
accessible to everyone, enabling parents to make informed choices.

National Childbirth Trust	Tel. 0870 770 3236 for enquiries
Alexandra House	Fax 0870 770 3237
Oldham Terrace	E-mail enquiries@national-childbirth-trust.
Acton	co.uk
London	http://www.nctpregnancyandbabycare.
W3 6NH	com

Nausea and vomiting

A mild condition common in early pregnancy / primigravidas – possibly debilitat-
ing (although a 'minor disorder').

Moderate / severe, i.e. hyperemesis gravidarum (hyper = excess; emesis =
vomiting; gravidarum = related to pregnancy).

Signs and symptoms:
Mild:

Commoner in the morning, particularly on waking, may last all day
Food / drink aversions, e.g. tea, coffee, fatty foods
Eating / drinking possible

Moderate / severe:

Continuous vomiting / no oral intake
Signs of dehydration, i.e. dry mouth / skin; ketonuria; oligouria (poor / no urine
output); halitosis (bad breath); sunken eyes.
Weight loss
Exhaustion
Drowsiness
Disorientation

Aetiology:

Not always clear-cut
Raised hormone levels, especially in early pregnancy

Oestrogen and hCG (human chorionic gonadotrophin from placenta)

Thyroid activity (severe cases)

Reduced gastric motility with / without reflux oesophagitis

Pre-eclampsia

Multiple pregnancy

Psychological factors, e.g. unwanted pregnancy (controversial)

Fetal genetic abnormality

Hydatidiform mole

Incidental conditions, e.g. infection (especially UTI); gastro-enteritis; peptic ulcer; hiatus hernia

Management
Mild:

Individual trial-and-error solutions

Small, frequent, light meals, avoiding spicy and fatty foods

Dry toast / biscuit before rising and frequently during the day

Soda water

Vitamin B_6 – avoid overdose

Ginger – biscuits, capsules, stem ginger

Complementary therapies, e.g. acupressure (sea bands for travel sickness), acupuncture or hypnotherapy; homeopathy (see Rule 7, NMC 2004b)

Moderate / severe:

Medical aid (Rule 6, NMC 2004b)

Admission to hospital

History

Observations – vital signs; fluid balance; urine output

Investigations, e.g. urinalysis / MSSU; infection screening; USS; FBC, Hb, U & E; IVI – Hartmann's solution or dextrose / glucose; ? added potassium

Antiemetic, e.g. prochlorperazine (Stemetil) or metaclopramide (Maxolon)

Basic nursing care

Oral fluids / light diet prn

Termination of pregnancy if improvement fails / condition becomes life-threatening

Neural tube defect (NTD)

A collective term for several central nervous system abnormalities, i.e.:

(i) anencephaly – absent skull vault / poor brain development (incompatible with life)

(ii) cerebral meningocele – involves the skull, commonly the posterior fontanelle

(iii) hydrocephalus – raised CSF causes large head

(iv) microcephaly – small skull vault, ? failed brain growth

(v) spina bifida – the spinal area

Aetiology:

Failed normal fetal growth

Linked to lack of folic acid before conception / during early fetal development

Microcephaly linked to intrauterine infection, e.g. rubella, toxoplasmosis

Genetic

Drugs, e.g. rifampicin (for TB)

Recognition:

Antenatal screening – blood for AFP; amniocentesis; USS

Initial neonatal examination

Neonatal USS

Hydrocephalus – wide bulging fontanelles

Prevention:

Avoid antenatal infection – rubella immunisation; effective hygiene, e.g. with cats

Routine folic acid 3 months pre-conception and first trimester

Management:

Early antenatal detection ? offer TOP

Neonatally depends on condition

Paediatric referral

Parental information / support

Complications:

Parental stress / anxiety, rejection

Hydrocephalus – CPD, obstructed labour; caesarean section

Increased infection risk

Long-term morbidity – physical, psychological, social for parents / child

Occipito-posterior (OP) position

A malposition of the occiput which lies in the posterior of maternal pelvis towards a sacro-iliac joint, either right (ROP) or left (LOP) or directly towards the sacrum (OP)

Aetiology:

Often unclear

Pelvic shape, e.g. android, anthropoid, flat sacrum

Pendulous abdomen
Anterior placenta

Diagnosis:
Pregnancy – alerting signs:
Abdomen appears flattened / slightly depressed below umbilicus
Fetal limbs on both sides
Back palpation difficult / impossible
FH heard just below umbilicus / on flank
Backache
Failed / late engagement of fetal head – wide presenting part (if deflexed head)
Prolonged discomfort under xiphisternum / breathlessness

Labour – alerting signs:
Abdominal examination
Suprapubic / back pain, especially during contractions
Excessively painful or poor contractions
Delayed head descent / advancement
Prolonged labour
VE:
      (i)   high presenting part
      (ii) cervix loosely applied, possibly oedematous
      (iii) slow, uneven cervical dilatation
      (iv) urge to push before cervix is fully dilated

Labour – confirming signs:
VE:
      (i)   anterior fontanelle either central or anterior
      (ii) posterior fontanelle possibly just tipped posterior
           (see Diagram 1.1)

Mechanisms:
Flexed head:
Lie longitudinal
Vertex presenting, flexed attitude
ROP or LOP position
Suboccipito-frontal diameter (10 cm) engages
As occiput reaches pelvic floor long rotation to OA occurs
Normal delivery (see Diagrams 1.2, 1.3)

Deflexed head:
Lie longitudinal
Vertex presenting

Military attitude

ROP / LOP

Occipito-frontal diameter (11.5 cm) engages

As descent takes place one of the following occurs:

    (i)   flexion occurs as above

    (ii) partial extension occurs – brow presents (no vaginal delivery)

    (iii) complete extension occurs – face presents

    (iv) if deflexed attitude persists:

        (a) sinciput reaches pelvic floor

        (b) short rotation (45°) of sinciput to anterior, direct OP

        (c) face to pubes delivery

            OR

        (a) occiput attempts long rotation to OA but

        (b) becomes caught on prominent ischial spines – deep transverse arrest

        (c) fetal head rotated using Kielland's forceps / Ventouse

        (d) head delivery using mid-cavity forceps, e.g. Simpson's, or Ventouse

Management – pregnancy:

May encourage anterior rotation of occiput / back by:

    periodically maintaining forward position, e.g. hands–knees, swimming

    lateral position for resting

    avoid prolonged, deep reclining position, e.g. on sofa, in bed, in car

Management – labour:

Close monitoring of progress

Information, support, encouragement

Leaning forward position / hands–knees position

Back massage ? relieves pain

Use bath / birthing pool, especially in hands–knees

Maintain empty bladder

Adequate analgesia – ? epidural

Augmentation of labour prn

Instrumental / operative delivery prn

Complications:

PROM (ill-fitting presenting part)

Prolapsed cord (ill-fitting presenting part)

Prolonged labour – first / second stages

Difficulty / inability PU

Premature pushing urge
Trauma – cervix, perineum
Instrumental / operative delivery
Fetal hypoxia
Excessive moulding of fetal skull
Birth trauma
Perinatal mortality
Long-term morbidity for mother / child
Psychological trauma / post-traumatic stress

Student activity:
Practice mechanisms with doll and pelvis
Simulated VE with OP positions
Further reading: Walmsley 2000

Ophthalmia neonatorum

Definition:
Purulent discharge from the eyes of the newborn within 21 days of birth

Signs:
Yellowish discharge from eye, commonly at 3–4 days
Inflamed / swollen eyelid
? Inflamed conjunctiva

Aetiology:
Infection e.g. *E. coli*, *Staphylococcus*, *Streptococcus*, gonorrhoea, *Chlamydia trachomatis* (occasionally none identified)
Poor infection resistance, e.g. prematurity, traumatic birth
Blocked tear ducts
Maternal genital tract infection
Cross-infection (including professionals!)
Poor hygiene

Prevention:
Recognition / treatment of maternal infection
Avoid contact with infected people
Effective hygiene, especially hand-washing
Minimal routine eye cleansing

Management:
Notify paediatrician (see activities of a midwife, *EU Second Midwifery Directive 80/155/EEC* in NMC 2004b)

Eye swab culture / sensitivity

Bathe eye with sterile water / cool boiled water at home – swab once inside to out (NB hand-washing!)

Chloramphenicol eye drops / ointment – ? before swab results

Tetracycline drops / ointment for *Chlamydia*

? Systemic antibiotics

Mother and partner treated if gonorrhoea / *Chlamydia*

ORACLE trial

Overview of the role of antibiotics in curtailing pre-term labour and early delivery. Begining in 1994, this international randomised controlled trial, funded by the Medical Research Council, aimed to see if treatment with broad-spectrum antibiotics would lessen neonatal mortality and morbidity due to PROM and pre-term birth.

Student activity:

Cross-reference PROM, pre-term labour, neonatal infections, maternal infections

Further reading: Kenyon 1995; Kenyon and Taylor 2002; King and Flenady 2002; Smaill 2001

Parent education

Can be:

Formal / informal

Planned / opportunistic

Individual / group sessions

Antenatal, intrapartum, postpartum

At home, in a community / hospital setting

NHS or private, e.g. National Childbirth Trust (NCT)

Before undertaking consider:

How people learn – active participation ('doing' / experiencing) aids learning

Why people learn – relevance to needs

When people learn: self-initiated learning lasts longer

Who learns:

mother, father, siblings, grandparents

the community (see activities of a midwife, *EU Second Midwifery Directive 80/155/EEC* in NMC 2004b)

People with special / additional needs:

(i) physical, sensory, learning disabilities

(ii) ethnic groups (especially if first language not English)

(iii) travellers

(iv) socio-economically / educationally disadvantaged / teenagers / substance-abusers

(v) what they might need to know / want to know

Aids to learning:

(i) non-threatening environment

(ii) mutual respect

(iii) enthusiasm

(iv) enjoyment

(v) variety of methods

(vi) topics selected by the group

Attention span (only 10–20 minutes) – therefore reinforce oral information with written

Student activity:

Note midwives' opportunities for offering individualised parent education.

Identify availability / format of sessions in your area (including private sector).

Are special / additional needs being catered for?

Consider your own educational needs in order to provide parent education.

Further reading: Schott 2002a,b; Walker and Pollard 1995; Whitton 1995

Partogram completion

Commenced when labour established – speedy reference to progress in chart form with common information:

Name, age, address, next of kin, religion, case sheet number

Special instructions

Routine observations recorded:

Temperature, pulse, blood pressure

Vaginal examinations – cervical dilatation, station of the head

Frequency / strength uterine contractions

Liquor / loss *per vaginam*

Reaction to pain

Drugs administered / method of analgesia

Student activity:

Familiarise yourself / practise completing partogram used in your unit

Further reading: Vincent 2003

Perineal repair (see perineal / surrounding area trauma below)

Part of a midwife's role (after instruction) to suture episiotomies / uncomplicated perineal tears – obstetrician's role if complicated – aseptic technique

Aim:

Ideally repaired promptly – secures homeostasis / prevents oedema / infection

Delay ? makes procedure more difficult

Minimise discomfort

Align tissues correctly

Reduce infection / deep vein thrombosis risk

Preparation:

Trolley with:

    (i)   appropriate instruments

    (ii) antiseptic solution

    (iii) local anaesthetic (see **episiotomy**, in Section 2 above, under anaesthetic, for perineal infiltration technique)

    (iv) suture materials – current evidence and research indicates polyglycolic acid Vicryl Rapide* causes less discomfort (Gemynthe *et al.* 1996)

Good light source

Explain procedure

Entonox available prn

Lithotomy poles

Stool for midwife to sit on whilst suturing

Woman – bladder empty / in lithotomy position

Maintain privacy

Action:

Midwife scrubs / wears sterile gloves

Vulva / perineum swabbed

Perineum re-infiltrated prn

Vagina examined – tear / episiotomy apex identified

? Vaginal swab / tampon inserted (maintains clear site)

Suture:

    (i)   beginning at apex – continuous suture to vaginal mucosa, knot tied aligning fourchette

    (ii) two / three interrupted sutures into deep perineal layers (avoiding rectal mucosa)

    (iii) interrupted / continuous subcuticular suture to skin

Remove swab / tampon

Ensure haemostasis

Gentle rectal examination to ensure mucosa not caught

Swab vulva / perineum
Dry pad applied
Legs gently lowered

Following suturing
Mother made comfortable
Repair explained
Contemporaneous records

Student activity:
Identify suture material used in your unit
Observe procedure
Further reading: Olah 1994; Baston 2004

Perineal / surrounding area trauma (see also **perineal repair** in
Section 2 above)
Pelvic floor / vulval area injury: spontaneous / surgical incision
First-degree tear (laceration):
    Shallow wound involving fourchette skin only
Second-degree tear:
    Skin and perineal muscle damage, possibly with deep muscles / vaginal
        mucosa involved
Third-degree tear:
    Damage extends to anal sphincter
Fourth-degree:
    Damage through sphincter into rectal mucosa
Vaginal wall:
    Commonly posterior wall – vaginal mucosa ? muscle, ? without skin
        damage
Labial tears:
    Superficial skin tears, often very painful
Clitoral tears:
    Uncommon – very painful
Cervical tears:
    Profuse bleeding likely
Episiotomy:
    A surgical incision of perineal skin, superficial / deep muscle, and vaginal
        mucosa, following local anaesthetic infiltration, enlarges vaginal orifice
        (opening).

Aetiology – tears:

Rapid, uncontrolled birth of baby's head (no gradual tissue stretching)
May occur with cephalic presentation or after-coming head of breech
Large baby / broad shoulders
Malpresentation, e.g. occipito-posterior
Hand involvement, i.e. baby's hand at face / shoulder widens shoulder diameter
Alternative positions for birth, e.g. 'all fours' (labial, anterior wall, clitoral tears)
Weak scar tissue (previous childbirth / cervical surgery)
Instrumental delivery

Indications for episiotomy:

To speed delivery in fetal / maternal distress when head on the perineum
Minimise intracranial trauma in prematurity / breech
Seriously delayed second stage (? rigid, poorly stretching perineum)
Reduces maternal effort in serious medical condition, e.g. cardiac disease
Prevention of trauma to previous surgery, e.g. pelvic floor / bladder repair
Maternal request

Prevention of trauma – antenatal:

Well-balanced, nutritious diet
Good hygiene
Early detection / treatment infection
Pelvic floor exercises
Complementary methods, e.g. oral arnica; massage with essential oils (see Rule
    7, NMC 2004b)

Prevention – labour:

Careful VEs – avoid over-stretching / trauma, e.g. from Amnihook during
    ARM
Non-directed pushing in second stage (not Valsalva manoeuvre)
Appropriate use / timing of episiotomy
Consider maternal position during second stage
Controlled delivery of the fetal head ('guarding the perineum') (see McCandlish
    1999; McCandlish *et al.* 1998 and HOOP study in Section 2 above)
Avoid prolonged second stage – 'prolonged' definition controversial
Skilled instrumental delivery

Management – initial:

First-degree / labial tears:
    Only sutured if bleeding / extensive
    Sutures cause discomfort

Second-degree / vaginal wall:
  Sutured following local anaesthetic (part of midwife's role)
  Medical aid if tear is very ragged / complicated.
  ? Non-suturing (see Clements and Reed 1999)
  Suture material – current evidence and research: Vicryl Rapide * less discomfort (Gemynthe *et al.* 1996)
Third- / fourth-degree:
  Medical aid – senior obstetrician and anaesthetist
  Repair in theatre under GA
  Prophylactic antibiotics
Clitoral tear:
  Medical aid – ? sutured
Cervical tear:
  Urgent medical aid – senior obstetrician and anaesthetist
  Suturing in theatre under GA
  Management of haemorrhage
Episiotomy:
  As for second-degree
  Discuss / obtain consent during pregnancy or early labour (prevent litigation / assault charge) – (see Dimond 2002 Chapter 7)
  Record keeping of discussions / reason for episiotomy

Management – postnatal:

Good hygiene facilitates healing
Treat infection
Oral analgesic prn – e.g. paracetamol / combination, e.g. co-proxamol
Stinging by urine – during micturition position change; warm water application, e.g. using a jug, shower spray or bidet; application of a barrier, e.g. Sudocrem or Vaseline (anecdotal evidence) – NB moist healing is faster than dry healing
Application of cold compresses (Steen 1999; Steen and Cooper 1998)
No consensus of evidence about other ways of aiding healing / relieving pain
Alternative therapies e.g. homeopathic, essential oils

Complications:

Infection / wound breakdown
Perineal pain / discomfort
Long-term morbidity
        (i)   pain and dyspareunia (painful intercourse)
        (ii) psychological trauma
        (iii) relationship difficulties

   (iv) rectocele – hernia (bulging) of rectum into vagina (weak muscles)

   (v) cystocele – hernia of bladder into vagina

   (vi) fistula – opening between vagina and bladder (vesico-vaginal); or vagina and rectum (recto-vaginal) leading to incontinence

Student activity:

Revise wound healing

Note local policies regarding episiotomy

Elicit midwives' skills in preventing perineal trauma

Further reading: Barwise 1998; Lavin and Smith 1996; Layton 2004; Lee 2002; Olah 1994; Parsons 1997; Premkumar 2005; Steen 1998; Steen and Cooper 1998; Sultan 1997; Webb 1992

Phenylketonuria (PKU) (see also **heel prick** in Section 2 above)

An inborn error of metabolism of the amino acid phenylalanine – high blood levels are toxic to developing brain tissue; the metabolite phenylpyruvic acid is present in the urine

Aetiology:

Genetically inherited, autosomal recessive: i.e. both parents carry an affected gene; incidence 1 : 10,000 births

Deficiency of enzyme phenylalanine hydroxylase, which converts phenylalanine to tyrosine (both needed for growth)

Diagnosis:

Guthrie or Scriver test or chromatography on peripheral blood (see **heel prick** in Section 2 above) as part of routine neonatal screening (with parental consent)

Fetal DNA testing if parents known carriers

Management:

Efficient screening system; result-monitoring part of local protocols

Specialist paediatric unit referral / specialist dietitian

Regular blood phenylalanine levels

Low phenylalanine diet, i.e. special infant formula + some breast milk / normal infant providing essential phenylalanine

Liaison with health visitor / GP

Phenylalanine-free supplements from weaning

'Special' low-protein foods available – bread, biscuits, flour, pasta

Measured everyday foods, e.g. cereal, milk, potatoes, provide essential phenylalanine

Genetic inheritance, e.g. PKU

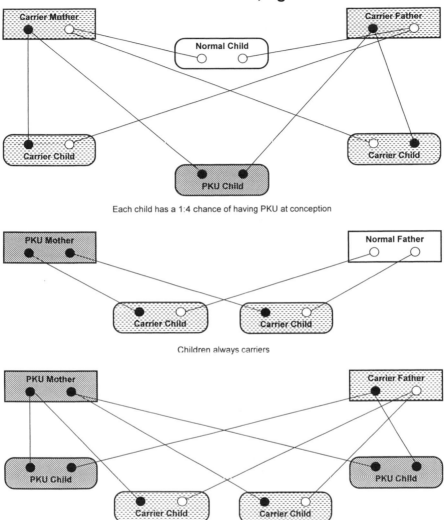

Figure 8 Genetic inheritance, e.g. PKU

Diet now recommended to continue for life
(NB women with PKU must resume very low phenylalanine diet six months
  before and throughout pregnancy, to avoid fetal brain damage)
Support from PKU society

Consequences – if untreated:
Growth retardation
Microcephaly
Brain damage
Eczema
Fair hair and skin very marked
Urine has 'mousy' smell

Student activity:
Note your local policy regarding routine screening, including other tests on the
same specimen
Further reading:
http://oxemedinfo.jr2.ox.ac.uk/Pathway/Disease/3305.htm
http://www.shsweb.co.uk/checklist/inborn/index.htm
http://www.shsweb.co.uk/check98/phlexy10sys.html
http://web.ukonline.co.uk/nspku/index/htm
http://www.kcl-phs.org.uk/haemscreening/newbornl.htm

PKU Society
A national support group for parents and children with PKU. Founded in 1973, it
is the oldest PKU support society in the world.

NSPKU	Tel. 0845 603 9136
PO Box 26642	email info@nspku.org
London N14 4ZF	http://nspku.org.uk

Phototherapy (see also **jaundice** in Section 2 above)
Treatment for physiological / prematurity jaundice, ABO incompatibility
Photoisomeration reduces jaundice – blue-spectrum light converts fat-soluble
bilirubin into less toxic water-soluble bilirubin for excretion
Equipment commonly administers white and blue light:
      (i)   Over the cot, portable light – baby's eyes covered
      (ii) Biliblanket – providing fibreoptic light – mat placed beneath / around
           baby – eyes uncovered / improved temperature maintenance

Aim:
Reduce serum bilirubin levels
Maintain body temperature
Prevent retinal damage
Reassure / support mother

Preparation:

Phototherapy unit at mother's bedside

Observation charts prn

Adequate room / incubator temperature (baby nursed naked – check body temperature)

Cover baby's eyes – secure eye pads, visor, shield over head

Action:

Baby naked under lights / on Biliblanket or Bilibed

Ensure adequate eye protection

Maintain observation chart

Check baby comfortable

Advise mother to remove baby for feeding, clean and undress, return

No creams – danger of burning

? Extra fluids during treatment

Bilirubin levels 8–12 hrly

Continue phototherapy 36–48 hrs

Note skin rashes / diarrhoea

When discontinued, continue bilirubin levels ? rise again

Record discontinuation

Student activity:

Further reading: Mills and Tudehope 2001; Pritchard *et al.* 2005

PIPPIN – Parents in Partnership Parent Infant Network

A national charity whose aim is to improve the emotional health of families at the time surrounding the birth of a baby. They also offer training courses for professionals.

Birch Centre Annex, Highfield Park,   tel. 01727 899099

Hill End Lane, St Albans, Herts. AL4 0RB   http://www.pippin.org.uk

Placental examination

Performed quickly initially at delivery, then in more detail once mother / baby comfortable

Aim:

Confirm placenta / membranes complete

Identify abnormality

Note number of placentae as potential indicator of zygosity in multiple births

Preparation:
Protected examining area
Midwife wears gloves / plastic apron
Good light source

Action:
Identify normality or anomalies
Examine fetal surface:
Note cord insertion – identify battledore / velamentous insertion
Check for three vessels
Note true / false knots
Note if bipartite
Examine placental circumference:
? Blood vessels into membranes / succenturiate lobes
Peel membranes apart, viewing amnion / chorion (amnion peels back to cord, chorion to placental edge)
Eliminate double chorion ring around circumference (circumvallate placenta)

Normal placentae:

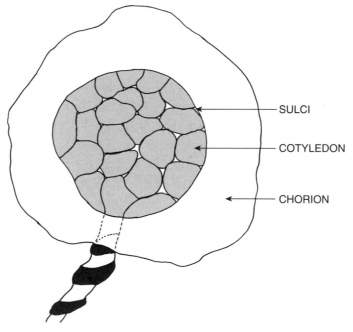

Diagram 5.1 Normal placenta at term – maternal surface
Note cotyledons, sulci, chorion

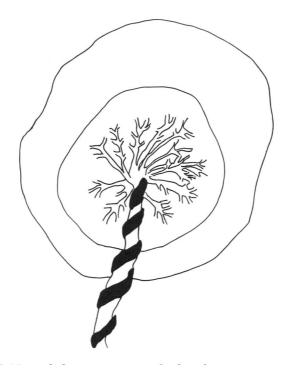

Diagram 5.2 Normal placenta at term – fetal surface
  Cord vessels supported by Wharton's jelly
  Two arteries and one vein twist around each other
  Vessels run deep into the placenta and extend over the surface

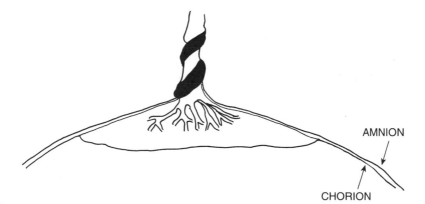

Diagram 5.3 Lateral view of placenta showing two membranes
  The chorion ends at the edge of the placenta
  The amnion peels back to the cord

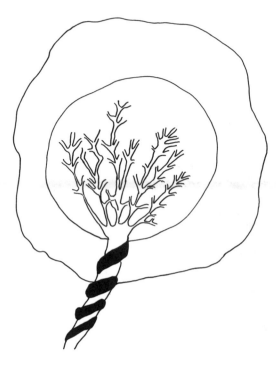

Abnormal insertions of the cord:

Diagram 5.4 Battledore insertion

Cord is inserted at the edge of the placenta

Danger of snapping during controlled cord traction (CCT)

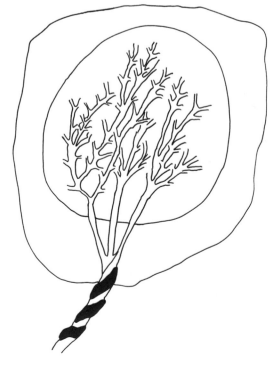

Diagram 5.5 Velamentous insertion

Vessels travel through the membranes to be inserted into the placenta

Danger of haemorrhage if the vessels lie over the cervical os (vasa praevia) and the membranes rupture

Membranes may tear and cord separate during CCT

Abnormal placentae:

Diagram 5.6 Succenturiate lobe of placenta

Blood vessels run through the membranes to an accessory lobe

Danger of haemorrhage from extra vessel if over cervical os (vasa praevia)

Extra lobe may not separate and be retained in utero

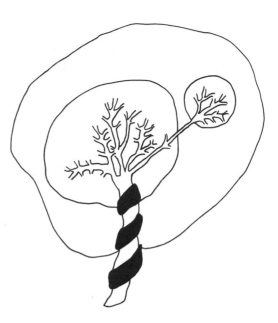

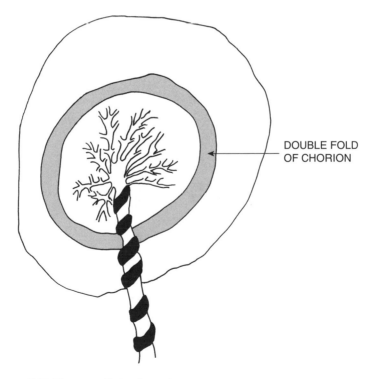

DOUBLE FOLD
OF CHORION

Diagram 5.7 Circumvallate placenta

Double fold of chorion around the circumference of the placenta apparent on the fetal surface as a thickened white ring

Associated with placental abruption

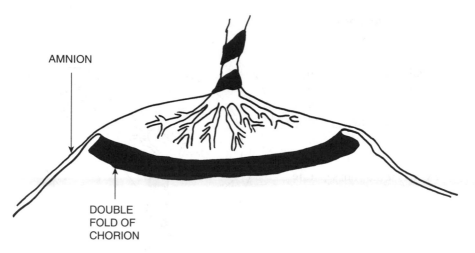

AMNION

DOUBLE
FOLD OF
CHORION

Diagram 5.8 Lateral view of circumvallate placenta showing the amnion and the double fold of the chorion

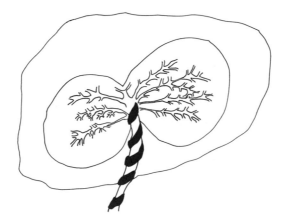

Diagram 5.9 Bipartite placenta
Two lobes of varying sizes with cord implanted between them
Danger of the cord snapping during CCT
One lobe may separate properly whilst the other is retained

Examine maternal surface:
    ? Normal colour / pale
    Consistency – ? normal, oedematous, calcification, 'grittiness', infarction
    Configuration – ? bipartite / tripartite
    ? Offensive
    Push cotyledons together – identify torn / missing pieces
Re-check chorion – ? extra lobes / holes

Multiple births

Two / more separate placentae examined as previously
If placentae fused together:
    ? Examination to determine if one placenta, i.e. monozygotic (uniovular) or
        > one, i.e. non-identical twins – dizygotic (binovular)
    Two amnions/ two chorions in twin pregnancy – ? = dizygosity (depends on
        when blastocyst divided)
    Method:
        (i) injecting fluid into cord and 'milking' it through placenta ? demon-
             strates whether the vessels go across – if yes, one placenta likely
             (monozygosity) – if no, two
        (ii) ? laboratory microscopic examination prn

Following examination

Dispose safely according to policy
If abnormality identified ? laboratory microscopic examination
If stillbirth – placenta to laboratory for further examination
Normal records

Student activity:

Seek every opportunity to examine placentae, especially if unusual
Further reading: Ventolini and Samlowski Hood 2004

Postnatal depression

A range of conditions, not always clearly defined or easily diagnosed, that include
    mild 'baby blues' (or 3rd / 4th day blues); depression; puerperal psychosis; and
    post-traumatic stress

Aetiology:

Not clear-cut – probably multifactorial
Previous psychiatric history
Existing neuroses, anxiety, phobia

Socio-economic problems:
- (i) relationship difficulties
- (ii) poor support
- (iii) unplanned / unwanted pregnancy
- (iv) major life events, e.g. bereavement / house move
- (v) financial / housing problems

Obstetric history:
- (i) loss previous pregnancy / baby
- (ii) complicated obstetric history
- (iii) difficult / traumatic pregnancy / birth (Crompton 1996; Laing 2001)
- (iv) a much-wanted pregnancy / baby – infertility treatment

Hormonal imbalance (Gregorie 1995) – history of PMT increases risk

'Baby blues':
Signs and symptoms:

Tiredness, weepy, feels emotionally low

Management:

Effective support
Rest / adequate sleep
Information / reassurance

Depressive illness:
Signs and symptoms:

Feelings of inadequacy / inability to cope
Crying / feeling very 'low'
Insomnia
Lack of feelings towards baby
Loss of libido
Severe tiredness not relieved by sleep / rest

Diagnosis:

Often difficult (Almond 1996) – reluctant admission to feeling unwell
Effective communication enables expression of feelings
Listen to relatives (? behaviour change noticed)
Edinburgh Postnatal Depression Scale (Webster *et al.* 2003) – 10 questions eliciting mother's feelings

Management: (Kumar *et al.* 1995; Hendrick 2003)

Give mother time to talk – effective listening skills
Debriefing of pregnancy and childbirth (present or past) experiences

Medical aid – ? antidepressants
Support from partner, relatives / significant person
? Postnatal support group
Quality rest and sleep
Alternative medicines (Mantle 2001)

Puerperal psychosis:
Signs and symptoms:
Obviously very ill
Altered perception of reality, e.g. of baby's abilities
Delusions, e.g. baby dead; not given birth
Confusion, e.g. about time / place
Hallucinations (auditory / visual)
Manic behaviour, e.g. obsessive cleaning
Insomnia

Management:
Medical aid and hospital admission to psychiatric ward – preferably with
baby
Sedation reduces symptoms, e.g. chlorpromazine
Appropriate treatment for diagnosis
? Electric convulsive treatment (ECT)
Promote mother–baby attachment and parenting ability – initial close
observation

Student activity:
Note your nearest psychiatric mother and baby unit
Further reading: Bott 1999a; Currid 2004; Davies 2003; Gaskell 1999; Gibbon
2004; Henderson *et al.* 2003; Hendrick 2003; Kennedy and MacDonald 2002;
Laing 2001; Robinson 1999; Sumner 2002

Postnatal exercises
Exercise sheets commonly available
Obstetric physiotherapist ? visit wards for support
Midwives' role to encourage frequent pelvic floor exercises

Aim:
Promote return of pelvic organs to pre-pregnancy state
Prevent thromboembolic disorders
Promote sense of well-being
Educate for future health

Preparation:
    Postnatal exercises sheet for referral
    Mother empties bladder
    Ensure privacy

Action:
    When recovered from delivery, encourage mobilisation
    Exercise gently initially – as strength returns, more vigorously
        (NB 3 months before progesterone effects subside)
    Feet – circular movements both directions; dorsiflex foot / wiggle toes
    Breathing – deep breathing / diaphragm used
    Pelvic floor – tighten vagina and rectum, hold for 10 seconds / release – repeat
        frequently when lying, sitting, standing
    Buttocks – clench / relax, simultaneous tightening pelvic floor – repeat
        frequently
    Hips – lying on bed, knees bent, feet to buttocks, swing knees side-to-side five
        times
    Back / abdomen – all fours, arch back (big curve) – hold a few seconds / relax
        / repeat
    Abdominal exercises – lying on back, knees bent, feet to buttocks – raise head
        / shoulders, touch right knee with left hand / hold / relax / repeat with other
        hand
    When standing – try lengthening leg by raising hip, repeat on other side

Student activity:
Identify local policy / practise yourself

Postnatal observations – baby (see **initial newborn examination** in
Section 2 above)

Aim:
    Detect deviation from normal – structure, function, behaviour
    Reassure mother of baby's progress
    Maintain accurate records

Preparation:
    Neonatal chart
    Explain procedure / seek consent
    Warm environment
    Wash hands beforehand or use gel substitute if hands clean

Action:

    Head – ? swellings, bruising, fontanelle tension

    Eyes – ? discharge

    Mouth – ? *Candida* (thrush) – white plaques on tongue not removable

    Facial skin – ? marks / pustules

    Ears – ? discharge

    Take axillary temperature / undress baby

    Body skin – ? rashes, pustules, blisters

    Colour – ? jaundice, cyanosis, pallor

    Umbilical cord – ? redness, stickiness, pus around base – if separated ? navel clean, dry, bleeding

    Buttocks / genitalia – ? rashes, redness, soreness

    Limbs – movement / position

    Note behaviour / muscle tone / reflexes

    Ask mother – about feeding, bowels, micturition, behaviour (fretful / distressed)

    Redress baby / give to mother

    Reassure mother by explaining findings

    Record accurately

Student activity:

Check local protocol for hand hygiene.

Revise neonatal thermoregulation.

Postnatal observations – mother

Maternal observations on ward admission / prior to leaving following home birth

Aim:

    Detect deviations from normal and seek medical aid (*Midwives' Rules and Standards* NMC 2004b)

    Early intervention preventing complications

    Advise woman of postnatal recovery

Preparation:

    Ensure privacy

    Postnatal records / charts available

    Explain examination / seek consent

    Woman lying almost flat

Action:

    Vital signs, i.e. TPR and BP prn

    Ask:

    (i)   how she is feeling / any concerns / coping

    (ii) about bowels / micturition – ? burning / stinging

    (iii) about sleep / appetite

    (iv) about lochia / breasts / pain

Check general appearance, colour, demeanour

Breast examination prn, e.g. nipples ? cracks / bleeding; engorgement, mastitis

Abdomen – palpate uterine fundus for consistency / position

Lochia – observe colour, odour, consistency (see BLiPP Study, Marchant *et al.* 1999 and 2000)

Perineal sutures – mother lateral position ? healing / infection

Legs – ? calf pain / tenderness, superficial phlebitis, oedema

Accurately record in case notes

Medical aid sought prn

With the new *Midwives' Rules and Standards* (NMC 2004b) there is the potential for midwives to continue visiting mothers and babies after the previous cut-off point of 28 days following delivery. This enables the vital continuity of carer to continue when complications are either present or have the potential to develop, e.g. postnatal depression. It also enables the midwife to conduct the six-week postnatal examination once confident and competent to do so following adequate preparation ('Responsibility and sphere of practice', *Midwives' Rules and Standards* (NMC 2004b)

Student activity:
Further reading: Albers 2000; Mitchell and Doyle 2002; Moyzakitis 2004; Thompson 2004; Ward and Mitchell 2004

Post-partum haemorrhage – primary
Aetiology:
Failed contraction and retraction of the uterine muscle (the living ligature) to stop bleeding from the placental site

Genital tract trauma from tear / cut, e.g. cervix, vagina, labia, clitoris, lower uterine segment, ruptured varicose vein

Predisposing factors:
Previous history:

Grand(e) multiparity

Over-distended uterus, e.g. multiple pregnancy, polyhydramnios, large baby

Retained products of conception – placenta, membranes or clots

APH

Anaemia

Pre-eclampsia / eclampsia

Inefficient uterine action / prolonged labour / oxytocic drugs in labour

Abnormal uterus, e.g. in shape or with fibroid(s)

Drugs, e.g. anaesthetics, tocolytics (uterine relaxants) in pre-term labour

Infection

Inversion of uterus

Mismanaged 3rd stage, e.g. inappropriate manual stimulation of uterus

Rapid uncontrolled delivery

Maternal expulsive effort (pushing) before cervix is fully dilated

Difficult instrumental delivery or before cervix is fully dilated

Episiotomy on a thick perineum

Prevention / minimise risks:

Treat anaemia, pre-eclampsia; prevent eclampsia, infection

Effective labour management when risks identified, e.g.:

    (i)   hospital birth

    (ii) blood to laboratory for save serum

    (iii) IV cannula inserted, ? IVI

    (iv) prevent prolonged labour, exhaustion, dehydration, full bladder

    (v) appropriate use of oxytocics, including in 3rd stage

    (vi) obstetric registrar at delivery

Management (see Figure 9, p. 178):

Complications of PPH

Anaemia

Shock / collapse – renal damage / failure, or Sheehan's syndrome (see below)

DIC

Psychological morbidity, e.g. post-traumatic stress (see **postnatal depression** in Section 2 above)

Death – see Lewis 2004

Student activity:

Further reading: Crafter 2002

Post-partum haemorrhage – secondary

Aetiology:

Retained products of conception, i.e. placenta or membranes

Retained blood clots

Infection

Fibroid(s)

Post-partum haemorrhage – primary

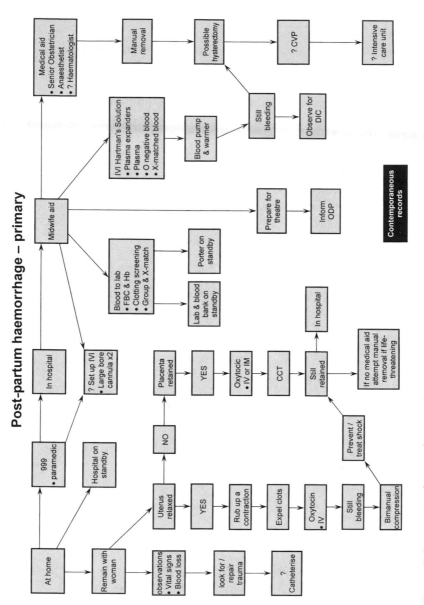

Figure 9 Post-partum haemorrhage – primary

Post-partum haemorrhage – secondary

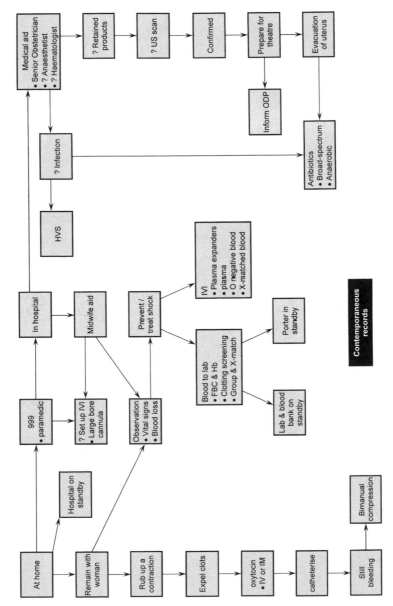

Figure 10 Post-partum haemorrhage – secondary

Signs and symptoms:
Subinvolution of uterus

Tender uterus

Lower abdominal pain / discomfort

Heavy lochia ? clots, membrane, placental tissue

Offensive lochia

Low grade pyrexia +/− tachycardia

General malaise (feeling unwell)

Management (see Figure 10, page 179):

Complications of PPH:
See above

Pregnancy-induced hypertension (PIH) and pre-eclampsia
Terms often used synonymously, but can be viewed as distinct

PIH:
Hypertension due to pregnancy, i.e. a BP of 140/90 or an increase in diastolic 15–20 mmHg above usual (e.g. booking recording) on 2 occasions 24 hours apart (NB – if diastolic normally 60, a rise to 80 is significant)

Pre-eclampsia:
Potential eclampsia (fulminating pre-eclampsia = eclampsia imminent)

No clear consensus on definition (Chappell *et al.* 1999; North *et al.* 1999; Steer 1999)

Commonly there is significant proteinuria (not due to UTI) and raised BP as above (NB eclampsia may occur with normal BP) and ? significant oedema (e.g. facial)

Onset:
Commonly > 32 weeks ? earlier; ? < 20 weeks if hydatidiform mole (see Section 1)

Condition variable in speed / progression

Aetiology:
Not clear-cut; associated with a gravid uterus – resolves after delivery

Possibly multifactorial / multi-system

Possibly superimposed on existing high BP

Hypotheses:
1. oxidative stress from high levels of circulating free radicals causing maternal vascular malfunction (Chappell *et al.* 1999)
2. placental influence
    (i) placental bed ischaemia, i.e. poor uterine artery flow, with high utero-placental resistance, due to poor implantation of trophoblast
    (ii) one or more factors from placenta transferred into maternal circulation, damaging blood vessels' endothelium; spasm raises BP; leaky vessels cause oedema
3. hormonal imbalance, e.g. prostaglandins
4. renin / angiotensin imbalance
5. immunological factors
    (i) commoner in primigravidas (sensitivity to 'foreign' genetic material)
    (ii) previous pregnancy (even aborted) offers some protection (sensitivity lowered)
    (iii) can occur (possibly for first time) if pregnant by new partner
6. maternal genetic factors – often familial, i.e. mother / sister had condition

Pre-disposing factors:

primigravida	grand(e) multigravida	multiple pregnancy
very young	>35	obesity
social class V	Rhesus isoimmunisaton	hydatidiform mole
diabetic	previous PIH/pre-eclampsia	? ethnicity

Management:
Prevention
? Low-dose aspirin (inhibits platelet aggregation in placental site) (see CLASP trial, Every 1994)

Dietary modification:
    (i) evening primrose oil or fish oil and / or calcium (balance prostaglandins) – inconclusive
    (ii) vitamin C 1000 mg + vitamin E 400 IU daily from early pregnancy (lowers circulating free radicals) – positive results from small pilot study of women at risk (Chappell *et al.* 1999)

Magnesium sulphate (see Duley *et al.* 2003; **MAGPIE trial** in Section 2 above)

Pregnancy
Regular monitoring of all women – they generally feel well until fulminating pre-eclampsia; therefore information to all women during pregnancy on recognition / action to take.

Diastolic <100 *no* proteinuria or symptoms:
rest at home, midwife checking BP and urine; ? self-monitoring
Diastolic <100 + proteinuria / symptoms:
admission
Diastolic >100 +/− proteinuria or symptoms:
admission

After admission:

Depends on severity of condition – intensive care may be needed (maternity unit / ICU)

Note general condition including temp. / pulse

BP 4- hourly or as frequently as every 15–20 min.

Fluid balance – particularly urine output ? catheterise (hourly measurement)

IVI, ? CVP, nil orally

Urinalysis for protein – ? 24-hour urine for total protein

MSSU to exclude UTI

Regular blood tests, e.g. 12–24 hours, for:
   (i)   FBC
   (ii) coagulation studies
   (iii) renal function – U & E; creatinine
   (iv) liver function – liver function tests, enzymes, AST (see Section 1)
   (v)   magnesium levels if administered (antidote calcium gluconate)

Control of BP, e.g.:
   (i)   methyldopa (Aldomet)
   (ii) labetolol
   (iii) hydralazine IM or IV for rapid control

Prevention of convulsions, e.g.:
   (i)   magnesium sulphate (Duley 1995; Lewis 1998, p. 45)
   (ii) phenytoin
   (iii) diazepam

Assess fetal well-being
   (i)   movements
   (ii) abdominal examination
   (iii) CTG daily
   (iv) US scans and biophysical profile

Labour / delivery

Induction of labour / caesarean section (NB clotting screening available)

Specific management if pre-term

Hospital (consultant unit) birth advisable – informed consent if woman wishes to remain at home (notify supervisor of midwives – see Rule 6, NMC 2004b)

Senior obstetrician / anaesthetist

Careful monitoring:

(i) hourly BP

(ii) continuous CTG

(iii) fluid balance (NB syntocinon anti-diuretic properties avoid fluid overload)

Adequate analgesia (epidural useful – lowers BP) to avoid stress from pain

Be prepared for possible complications, e.g.:

(i) ? haematologist / blood lab. on standby

(ii) drugs / equipment available

(iii) paediatrician at delivery or on standby

(iv) ? neonatal unit on standby

Syntocinon for 3rd stage (not Syntometrine – vaso-constriction effect of ergometrine increases BP)

Postnatal

Continue observation of BP (haemoconcentration may cause rise in BP)

Eclampsia risk for 48 hours

? Continue antihypertensives

Complications:

Fulminating pre-eclampsia = imminent eclampsia

Recognition:

Headaches, retinopathy, visual disturbances

Renal damage

(i) proteinuria

(ii) oligouria

(iii) raised blood urea

Hepatic damage

(i) abdominal / epigastric pain (blood under liver capsule)

(ii) vomiting (NB ? misdiagnosing less serious conditions)

(iii) jaundice – raised liver enzymes and AST (see Section 1)

Thrombocytopenia – i.e. low platelets due to consumption – possible DIC

Haemolytic anaemia

HELLP syndrome

(i) **H**aemolysis

(ii) **E**levated **L**iver enzymes

(iii) **L**ow **P**latelets (Nutt 1997; Sibai 2004a)

Placental abruption / APH – possible DIC

Myocardial infarction (heart attack)

CVA (cerebro-vascular accident – stroke)

Adult RDS

Eclampsia

Death:
See *Why Mothers Die 2000–2002* (Lewis 2004)

Mid trimester miscarriage

Placental insufficiency (nutrient and O_2 deficiency) leading to IUGR; fetal hypoxia; IUD

Pre-term delivery

Perinatal death

Student activity:
Revise normal BP regulation mechanisms / changes antenatally
Note non-pregnancy causes of hypertension
Note your local management policies for PIH / pre-eclampsia
Further reading: Draycott *et al.* 2000; Duley *et al.* 2003; McDonald 2002; Morley 2004; Roberts 1999

Pre-labour or premature rupture of membranes (PROM)
(see also **pre-term labour** and **pre-term baby** below)

Incidence:
Approximately 2–17% – many cases ? unrecognised

Aetiology:
Unclear – known risk factors
Previous history PROM
Cervical surgery, e.g. cone biopsy
Unhealthy placenta
Antenatal procedures, e.g. amniocentesis

Uterine trauma

Lower genital tract infections, e.g. *Trichomonas*, group B strep., *Staphylococcus aureus*, Group B strep. in previous child

ECV

Smoking

Hypertensive disorders

Diabetes

Malpresentation

? Coitus (? due to prostaglandins in semen / released from cervix)

? VE

? Other genital tract infections, e.g. gonorrhoea, yeasts (thrush), *Chlamydia*

Management:

History:

Onset of loss, amount, colour, smell, blood

Differentiate with incontinence of urine / leucorrhoea

Gestation, LMP / USS

Risk factors present

Present symptoms:

General condition, including pyrexia

Vaginal loss

Contractions

Dysuria

Other symptoms

Social situation – help / support needed enabling rest

Examinations:

General condition and vital signs

Abdominal palpation

Auscultation FH

CTG

?Speculum VE for: (NB *no* digital VE until labour begins – infection risk)

    (i)   cervical and low vaginal swabs

    (ii) confirmation liquor present, ? nitrazine stick (not 100% reliable)

    (iii) note cervical dilatation

USS:

    (i)   biophysical profile

    (ii) abnormalities

(iii) gestation

(iv) weight estimation

If 37 weeks or more and no complications / risk factors:

(i)   ? await onset of labour (24–48 hrs.)

(ii) ? go home / return daily for review

(iii) ? immediate induction or wait 24–48 hrs. (Syntocinon or vaginal Prostin)

(NB – woman's informed choice – risk of infection rises >24 hrs.)

If mother / baby at risk whatever gestation – expedite delivery

If pre-term PROM (i.e. before 37 weeks):

(a) senior obstetric / paediatric medical aid

(b) *if* 32 weeks or less, or baby estimated <2500 g, and delivery expected – mother in unit with NNICU (possible *in utero* transfer, i.e. of pregnant woman to appropriate unit)

(c) *if* fetus not compromised, and delivery not expected – treat conservatively:

(i)   maternal rest – hospital

(ii) observe for infection:

- general condition
- vital signs
- blood for white cell count and ESR daily
- fetal tachycardia (reliable >28 weeks)

(iii) CTG daily

(iv) ? tocolytics (inhibit contractions) – useful for *in utero* transfer

(v) ? antibiotics (controversial), e.g. ampicillin / penicillin G, IM, or erythromycin

(vi) ? home if liquor lessens – continue monitoring / screening

(d) *if* 24–34 weeks / delivery expected, IM corticosteroids – see **pre-term labour** below

Complications:

Cord prolapse leading to:

Hypoxia / birth asphyxia

Perinatal death

Long-term morbidity, e.g. cerebral palsy

Social / psychological trauma

Intrauterine infection leading to:

IUD

Maternal infection / puerperal sepsis

Maternal / neonatal mortality / morbidity

Social / psychological trauma

Student activity:

Note your local policy and procedures

Further reading: Kenyon 1995; Kenyon *et al.* 2004; Smaill 2001

Pre-term baby (see also **small for gestational age baby (SGA)** and **pre-term labour** below)

A baby born <37 completed weeks gestation – may also be small for gestational age (SGA)

      (i)   low birth weight <2500 g

      (ii) very low birth weight <1500 g

      (iii) extremely low birth weight <1000 g

Characteristics:

Head:

Appears large in proportion to baby

Fontanelles / sutures wide

Skull bones soft

Eyelids ? fused

Pinna of ear soft / will remain folded

Length:

Proportional to weight

Limbs:

Thin

Nails soft, usually short

Muscle tone:

Poor

Arms / legs abducted

Chest:

Small and narrow

Little / no breast tissue

Skin:

Red / pink, transparent – veins visible

Lacks subcutaneous fat

Lanugo (hair) present, depending on gestation

Vernix often marked, depending on gestation

Abdomen:
Large
Umbilicus may appear low

Genitalia:
Small
Testes may be undescended
Labia majora not covering minora

Behaviour:
Cry weak / absent
Little activity
Poor / no sucking / swallowing

Aetiology:
Often unknown
Spontaneous / induced for maternal condition
Pre-eclampsia / hypertensive disease
APH
Maternal disease, e.g.:
  (i)   renal
  (ii) diabetes
  (iii) severe infection, especially UTI, including asymptomatic bacteruria
Cervical incompetence
Smoking, drug, alcohol abuse
Multiple pregnancy
Polyhydramnios
Rhesus incompatibility
Higher incidence in:
  (i)   malposition / malpresentation
  (ii)   teenage pregnancy
  (iii) multiparas
  (iv)   poor maternal nutrition
  (v)   low socio-economic groups
  (vi)   psychological factors, e.g. stress and anxiety; violence and abuse
  (vii) abnormal uterus, e.g. bicornuate
  (viii) repeated TOP – ? damaged uterus / cervix
  (ix)   abdominal surgery, e.g. appendectomy; removal ovarian cyst

Management – initial (see also **pre-term labour** below)

Delivery in consultant unit with NNICU (? *in utero* transfer – trained escort)

Paediatrician at delivery

Necessary resuscitation measures (see **birth asphyxia** in Section 2 above)

Maintain body temperature (see **hypothermia – neonatal** in Section 2 above)

Initial parent–baby contact

Transfer to NNICU

Assessment of gestational age (see **Dubowitz Score** in Section 1)

Weigh and place in incubator

Base-line observations via monitoring equipment:

      (i)   temperature

      (ii) respiratory rate and oxygen saturations

      (iii) heart rate

      (iv) blood glucose (see **heel prick** in Section 2 above)

? IVI +/or arterial line (usually umbilical artery via cord stump)

? Intubation and ventilation

? Infection screening

? Prophylactic antibiotics

Information and support to parents

Management – subsequent:

(NB – may involve moral / ethical dilemmas for parents / staff – support essential)

Maintain respiration / oxygen levels

Monitor vital signs

Thermoregulation (see **hypothermia – neonatal** in Section 2 above)

Monitor / maintain blood glucose

Fluid balance

Hygiene and prevention of infection

Feeding:

      (i)   parenteral (IVI)

      (ii) enteral (into gut via oral / naso-jejunal tube)

      (iii) intragastric (oral / naso-gastric tube)

      (iv) oral

Parental information / psychological support

Parental participation in care encouraged

Consider individual cultural, religious, personal beliefs / values and needs

Paediatric follow-up after discharge

Complications:
 Perinatal / neonatal death
 Associated with specific congenital abnormalities
 Birth asphyxia
 Cerebral haemorrhage
 Persistent fetal circulation
 RDS / SDS (surfactant deficiency / respiratory distress syndrome)
 Hypothermia
 Hypoglycaemia
 Hypocalcaemia
 Jaundice
 Infection
 Anaemia
 Haemorrhagic disease
 Iatrogenic conditions (i.e. those due to treatment):
  (i) retinopathy
  (ii) bronchopulmonary dysplasia (BPD) – chronic respiratory disease (mechanical ventilation)
  (iii) necrotizing enterocolitis (NEC) – bowel inflammation, ischaemia and obstruction
 Long-term morbidity:
  (i) cerebral palsy
  (ii) motor / neurological impairment
  (iii) learning difficulties
 SIDS – increased risk

Student activity:
Revise fetal circulation / adaptation to extra-uterine life
Compare / contrast characteristics of pre-term / SGA baby
Further reading: Curran *et al.* 1997; Fraser and Cooper 2003, Chapter 41

Pre-term labour (see also **pre-labour or premature rupture of membranes (PROM)** and **pre-term baby** in Section 2 above)
Labour commencing <37 completed weeks gestation

Aetiology:
 Spontaneous – see **pre-term baby** in Section 2 above
 Induced for:
  (i) fetal compromise
  (ii) IUD
  (iii) maternal condition (see **induction of labour – alternative and natural**; and **induction of labour – medical** in Section 2 above)

Prevention:
Optimise maternal well-being – pre-conception and antenatal:
- (i) nutritious diet
- (ii) socio-economic factors
- (iii) infection screening and treatment for asymptomatic bacteruria (NICE 2003)
- (iv) management of maternal conditions
- (v) family spacing
- (vi) stop smoking / substance use

? Cervical suture for incompetent cervix

Management:
Admit to consultant unit with NNICU (? *in utero* transfer – trained escort)

Obstetric medical aid (senior)

History:
- (i) booking and antenatal
- (ii) gestation
- (iii) present general condition – including signs of infection
- (iv) vital signs
- (v) contractions
- (vi) vaginal loss

Examinations:
- (i) abdominal
- (ii) FH auscultation, CTG (min. 30 min.)
- (iii) ? digital VE by obstetrician if membranes intact
- (iv) speculum VE by obstetrician if membranes ruptured (see **pre-labour or premature rupture of membranes (PROM)** in Section 2 above)
- (v) urinalysis – routine dip stick and MSSU
- (vi) blood – FBC, ? group / save serum
- (vii) ? USS

Treat underlying cause

? Prophylactic antibiotics (see **ORACLE trial** in Section 2 above)

IVI – sodium lactate (Hartmann's solution) – rapid hydration ? decreases contractions

If 24–34 weeks and no contraindications:
- (a) IM corticosteroids to mature fetal lungs:
  - (i) dexamethasone 6 mg IM × 4 doses 12 hrs. apart; or
  - (ii) betamethasone 12 mg IM × 2 doses 24 hrs. apart (NB blood glucose levels will significantly rise in diabetics)
- (b) deliver in unit with NNICU (? *in utero* transfer – trained escort)

If no contraindications, e.g. compromised fetus, severe vaginal bleeding and 24–34 weeks – delay delivery long enough for corticosteroids to be effective – ? tocolytics (controversial), e.g.:

Tocolytic	Admin. route	Possible side-effects
(a) Ritodrine (Yutopar)	IVI	tachycardia and palpitations vomiting, headache tremors, anxiety
(b) Salbutamol (Ventolin)	IVI	tachycardia and palpitations vomiting, headache tremors, anxiety
(c) Terbutaline	SC / IVI	tachycardia and palpitations vomiting, headache tremors, anxiety
(d) Magnesium sulphate (calcium gluconate antidote)	IV bolus / IVI	resp. arrest in high doses neuromuscular effects monitor serum calcium and magnesium levels
(e) Indomethacin (inhibits prostaglandins)	oral / rectal	gastro-intestinal irritant headaches and dizziness ?closure of fetal ductus arteriosus
(f) Nifedipine (effective in prolonged use)	oral	facial flushing, headaches, oedema, constipation, hypotension

Complications:

Pre-term baby

Instrumental / operative delivery (short- and long-term maternal consequences)

Social and psychological implications

Student activity:

Revise the initiation of labour

Note your local policy and protocols

Further reading: Kenyon 1995; Smaill 2001

Primary Care Trusts (PCTs)

The PCTs replaced primary care groups. They are responsible for improving public health at local level by planning and commissioning health services. This includes ensuring that adequate staff and services are available from hospital and community services. This incudes GPs, dentists, mental health care, Walk-In Centres, NHS Direct, patient transport (including emergency), population screening, pharmacy and opticians. The integration of health and social care systems is included in their role.

Student activity:

Consider the role of the midwife in public health. Further reading: Edwards *et al.* 2005

Prolonged labour – first stage

There is no consensus of opinion about time, but commonly 12–24 hours in established labour (NB – avoid including time during the latent phase of the first stage) is considered prolonged.

Aetiology:

Inefficient / incoordinate uterine action

Malposition / malpresentation

CPD

Non-engagement of presenting part

Cervical dystocia, e.g. due to scarring from surgery or TOP

Psychological factors leading to hormonal / chemical imbalance, e.g. oxytocin and catecholamines

Entering birthing pool too early, e.g. before cervix 4–5 cm dilated

Management:

Identify possible cause

Mobility and upright position

Psychological support

Adequate analgesia

General physical care

Observations:
1. fluid balance
2. vital signs
3. urinalysis
4. progress:
    (i) contractions
    (ii) descent of presenting part – abdominally / on VE
    (iii) cervical dilatation

? continuous electronic monitoring
Augmentation / acceleration of labour as appropriate
Caesarean section as appropriate, e.g. for CPD

Complications:

Maternal stress:
    Anxiety
    Frustration
    Anger
    Tiredness or exhaustion
    Emotional
    Greater pain sensitivity
Maternal distress:
    Physical and emotional exhaustion
    Raised temperature and BP
    Dehydration and oligouria
    Ketosis
    Vomiting
Intrauterine infection
Ruptured uterus
Risk operative / instrumental delivery
Risk PPH
Fetal hypoxia
Early neonatal infection
Perinatal mortality
Neonatal / infant morbidity
Post-traumatic stress / long-term psychological trauma

Prolonged labour – second stage

Without progress in the active stage:
    >30 minutes for multipara
    >1 hour for primigravida
The timing is traditional, but debatable; a longer time is increasingly acceptable if fetal and maternal conditions are satisfactory and progress is being made.

Aetiology:

Inefficient uterine action
Poor maternal effort due to:
        (i)   exhaustion
        (ii) epidural
        (iii) fear / pain

Full rectum / bladder
Rigid perineum
Contracted pelvic outlet / CPD
Persistent OP position
Deep transverse arrest
Malpresentation

Management:

Support and encouragement
Change in maternal position, e.g.:

(i)   left lateral
(ii) upright
(iii) 'all-fours'

Close observation of FH (minimum every 5 min. – ? continuous)
Medical aid:

(i)   obstetrician
(ii) paediatrician
(iii) anaesthetist

Syntocinon infusion
? Episiotomy
? Instrumental delivery – forceps or ventouse
? Caesarean section

Student activity:

Note your local policies on definitions and management of prolonged labour

Pruritus

Itching – abdominal, vulval, general

Aetiology:

Abdominal:

Unclear
General skin stretching
Striae gravidarum, i.e. pregnancy stretch marks
Hormone links, e.g. corticosteroids

Vulva:

Infection, e.g. yeasts, i.e. *Candida* (thrush); bacteria
Sweat rash
Glycosuria

General:
  Allergic reaction – food; antibiotics; blood transfusion
  Infection, e.g. viral rash
  Cholestasis

Management:
Abdomen:
  Little effective prevention
  Moisturising cream popular
  Oil-based calamine lotion if severe

Vulva:
  Identify organism – HVS; vulval swab; and appropriate treatment
  Effective hygiene
  Urinalysis / investigate glycosuria
  Cotton underwear
  Avoid tights / tight-fitting clothes

General:
  Identify cause
  Withdraw allergen
  Antihistamine for allergic reactions
  Investigate possible cholestasis
  Local preparations to relieve itching, e.g. calamine lotion

Pudendal nerve block
  Pudendal nerves supply external genitalia, perineum, lower vagina
  Obstetrician's role ? prior to instrumental delivery / perineal repair
  Not always effective
  Transvaginal approach common – ischial spines are palpated / injection either
    side
  Perineal approach if presenting part very low

Aim:
  Assist the doctor
  Support woman / partner
  Maintain accurate records

Preparation:
  Delivery trolley with pudendal block pack (includes guarded needle, e.g. Oxford
    needle)

Local anaesthetic, e.g. lignocaine 0.5% / 1.0%
Syringes
Empty bladder
Entonox available

Action:

Explain procedure
Assist opening packs / drawing up local anaesthetic
Place legs in lithotomy position
Offer Entonox / support
Safely dispose of needles on completion
Ensure records completed

Pulse taking

Aim:

Palpate / count peripheral pulse (commonly radial; ? temporal)
Accurately record

Preparation:

Explain procedure
Client seated / resting
Watch / clock with second hand
Observation chart / records

Action:

Lift arm / place two fingers over wrist's inner border
Locate pulse / count for one minute
Note rate, if irregular, weak, bounding – record
Inform client of findings
Medical aid if abnormal

Relaxation techniques

Encouraged / practised during pregnancy since 1930s – Grantley Dick-Reid
proposed that stress / tension increased labour pain, causing more stress /
tension; but relaxation exercises break cycle – also information reduced fear
/ tension
Psychoprophylaxis – a series of relaxation / breathing exercises
Relaxation exercises helping us cope with everyday living can be beneficial in
pregnancy / labour

Aim:

Encourage total body relaxation during pregnancy

Increase body awareness

Provide sense of well-being / confidence

Preparation:

Small group teaching ideal

Mats / pillows

Advised loose clothing

Maintain privacy

Woman lying comfortably supported by pillows

Action:

Working from head to toes encourage awareness of posture / tension present, e.g.:

head – jaw tension

frowning – conscious effort to smooth brow

relax jaw

tongue comfortable in mouth / teeth not grinding.

neck – relaxed, head supported by pillows

shoulders – note tension, relax / let pillows support

arms – note muscle tension, let arms fall loosely by sides

hands – let fingers relax, palms open, wrists loose / floppy

legs / feet the same

abdominal muscles – relaxed buttocks / pelvic floor

total body relaxation

Encourage concentration on breathing; note different levels, i.e.:

deep breathing using diaphragm

shallow breathing using intercostal muscles

panting using upper respiratory muscles

Practise deep breathing / total relaxation – maintain awareness of feeling of full relaxation

Gradually increase body tension / return to sitting position / upright position

Student activity:

Attend local session / practice exercises

Respiratory distress syndrome (RDS) (Surfactant Deficiency Syndrome)

Respiratory condition – alveoli inflation difficult / impossible

commoner in neonate than adults

Neonatal

Aetiology:

Lack of surfactant (surface activating or active agent) causes alveoli to collapse on expiration, requiring great respiratory effort for the next breath – lecithin and sphingomyelin are precursors to surfactant, and can be measured antenatally in the liquor.

Predisposing factors:

Prematurity, especially <34 weeks:

Caesarean section

APH

Diabetic mother

Hypoxia / acidosis

Maternal drug abuse

Prevention

Delay pre-term delivery until lungs mature

Promote lung maturity / surfactant production – maternal IM dexamethasone or betamethasone (corticosteroids) (see **pre-term labour** in Section 2 above)

Avoid perinatal hypoxia / acidosis

Tight control on maternal diabetes antenatally

Control maternal drug addiction

Signs:

Difficulty initiating normal respiration

Breathing difficulties in first few hours after birth

Grunting sound on expiration

Hypotonia (poor muscle tone)

Sternum / intercostal muscles drawn in; flaring of nostrils

Cyanosis

Tachycardia

Reduced breathing sounds

X-ray picture

Management:

Paediatrician

Admission to NNICU

Intubation / mechanical ventilation

Monitor / maintain blood gases; temperature; blood glucose levels

Replacement surfactant therapy (Greenough 1997, Stevens *et al.* 2005)

Parental information / support

Complications:

Cerebral haemorrhage
Pneumothorax (air in chest cavity)
Persistent fetal circulation
Sepsis
DIC
Death
Long-term morbidity, e.g. broncopulmonary dysplasia (BPD) (long term O_2 need)
Neurological disorders

Adult:
Aetiology:

Profound hypoxia – hypotension; haemorrhage; DIC
Mendelson's syndrome
Hypertensive disorders
Sepsis

Management:

Medical aid – senior obstetrician / anaesthetist
Treat underlying cause
Assisted ventilation
Intensive care unit

Complications:

Maternal death – 44 direct deaths during 1988–90 (Hibbard *et al.* 1994)
Long-term physical, social, psychological morbidity

Student activity:

Further reading: Hibbard *et al.* 1994 Annexe to Chapter 9 Adult Respiratory Distress Syndrome, pp. 97–9; Lewis 2004

Resuscitation of newborn – see **birth asphyxia** in Section 2 above

Retained placenta (see **delivery technique** (third stage of labour) in Section 2 above)
The placenta is considered retained:

(i)   after 30 minutes in active 3rd stage
(ii) after 1 hour in physiological 3rd stage

It may be:

(i)   wholly or partially separated – danger of PPH

(ii) trapped in the cervix or uterus – danger of PPH

(iii) still adherent to the uterus – PPH less likely

Aetiology:

Uterine inertia:

(i)   failure of contraction and retraction of myometrium to separate and expel placenta

(ii) may follow incoordinate uterine action, prolonged or precipitate labour

Full bladder:

inhibits uterine function and/or delays descent of placenta

Mismanagement of 3rd stage:

(i)   use of CCT before Syntometrine is effective

(ii) 'fiddling' with the uterus – causes inertia or incoordinate uterine action

(iii) delay in using CCT following Syntometrine – causes placental entrapment by closed cervix

Uterine abnormality: e.g. bicornuate uterus increases risk.

Constriction ring – spasm of uterine muscles above lower segment inhibits expulsion.

Pre-term labour – particularly if induced

Adherent placenta:

(i)   partially, e.g. by infarcts

(ii) partially / wholly due to being:

(a) attached *to* myometrium (placenta accreta)

(b) attached *into* myometrium (placenta increta)

(c) attached *through* myometrium (placenta percreta)

Management (see Figures 11.1, 11.2 on pp. 202–3):

Manual removal:

An obstetric procedure, may be undertaken by a midwife in an emergency (see activities of a midwife, *EU Second Midwifery Directive 80/155/EEC* in NMC 2004b)

Morbidly adherent placenta may be retained for natural absorption

Complications

Post-partum haemorrhage

DIC

Retained placenta – at home

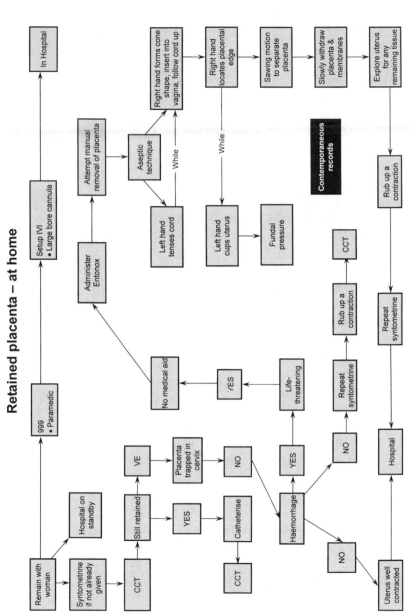

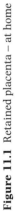

Figure 11.1 Retained placenta – at home

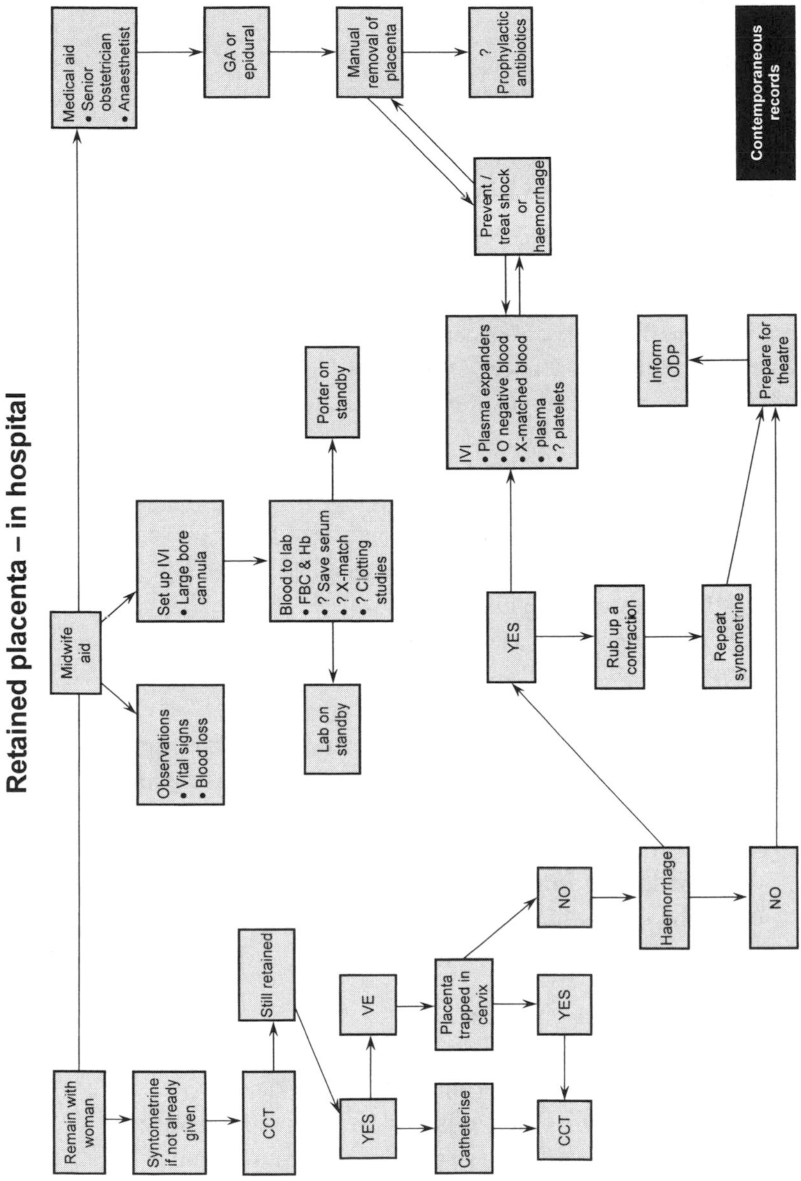

Retained placenta – in hospital

Figure 11.2 Retained placenta – in hospital

Perforated uterus

Sepsis

Death

Hysterectomy (especially if morbidly adherent) / subsequent infertility

Student activity:

Note your local policy / procedures for management in community / hospital
settings.

Retinopathy of the newborn (retrolental fibroplasia)

Abnormal development of blood vessels in the eye, which may regress or lead to
local or complete retinal detachment, with long-term consequences of visual
impairment or blindness.

The condition has five stages, from demarcation of vascular and avascular zones
to complete retinal detachment. Additional blood vessel abnormalities and
clouding of the vitreous humour, called plus disease, increase the severity of
the condition.

Aetiology:

Not fully understood – ? multifactorial

Pre-term / very low birth weight babies susceptible

Noted in stillborn / full-term infants

Oxygen therapy implicated, i.e. when levels too high, particularly in premature
infants

Hypothetical causes:

(i) toxic oxygen – O_2 therapy combined with blood transfusion / iron
neonatal hypoxia / anoxia, e.g. in bradycardia / apnoea

(ii) intrauterine hypoxia, e.g. in pre-eclampsia

(iii) intraventricular haemorrhage at delivery or after birth

(iv) inability to synthesise prostaglandins – linked to toxic oxygen

(v) light, e.g. 24-hour brightness while in incubator

Prevention:

Minimise risk of hypoxia / trauma

Avoid prematurity

Strict neonatal blood gas monitoring / control of O_2 levels

Reduce / discontinue O_2 as soon as possible – avoid rapid change

Minimal handling / procedures avoids O_2 concentration change

Rapid response to bradycardia / apnoea

Management:

Early screening by opthalmologist

Laser therapy or cryotherapy to minimise the destructive consequences of the
   condition
Paediatric follow-up

Complications:
Visual impairment, e.g. tunnel vision, due to:
   (i)   damaged retina
   (ii) retrolental (behind lens) fibrous mass
   (iii) cataracts; glaucoma
Myopia (short sight)
Nystagmus (rapid eye movements)
Strabismus (squint)
Photophobia (sensitivity to light)
Microphthalmia (small eyes)
Blindness

Student activity:
Further reading: Clarkson 2001, 2002

Safe Motherhood Initiative
With the aim of reducing world-wide maternal mortality and morbidity, the World
   Health Organisation (WHO) launched the Safe Motherhood Initiative in 1987.
   Key target areas are improvement in education / social standing for women;
   improvement in health services, including family planning; better education
   for midwives (especially untrained traditional birth attendants (TBA)), including how to manage emergency situations, e.g. PPH, eclampsia, and obstructed
   labour. Individual countries employ specific solutions to meet their unique
   needs.

Sexually transmitted diseases / infections (STDs / STIs) (see
also **antenatal screening** and **infection – maternal** and **infection –
neonatal** in Section 2 above)

Diseases spread by sexual contact:
Viral, e.g. hepatitis A, B, C; human papilloma virus (genital warts); *Herpes simplex*
   type 2; HIV
Bacterial, e.g. gonorrhoea; *Gardnerella*
Protozoal, e.g. *Trichomonas vaginalis*
Spirochaete, e.g. syphilis
Parasitic, e.g. *Chlamydia trachomatis*
Fungal (yeasts), e.g. *Candida* (thrush)

Sheehan's syndrome
Hypopituitarism, i.e. poor / failed pituitary function

Aetiology:
A rare anterior pituitary necrosis following prolonged shock (APH / PPH)

Signs and symptoms:
History
Failed lactation
Secondary amenorrhoea, i.e. no menstruation following childbirth
Diminished thyroid / adrenal function (lethargy, feeling cold, coarse skin / hair)
Libido loss
Diminished secondary sexual characteristics

Management:
Hormone replacements – thyroxin; corticosteroids; HRT

Complications:
Infertility – associated with hormone reduction / failure

Shoulder dystocia
A complex clinical phenomena (Mortimore and McNabb 1998)
An obstetric emergency – no classic definition:
Failure of spontaneous vaginal delivery of fetal shoulders after head has born (without use of specific manoeuvres) – commonly, anterior shoulder is obstructed behind the symphysis pubis / posterior shoulder below sacral promontory

Risk factors:
Large fetus – especially >4000 g – may be influenced by:
  (i) maternal age >35
  (ii) large maternal birth weight (not usually enquired about at booking)
  (iii) maternal obesity
  (iv) diabetes (gestational or existing) often causes macrosomic baby i.e. >4000 g

Pelvic abnormalities:
  (i) narrow outlet
  (ii) platypelloid shape
  (iii) small pelvis

Maternal immobility / position in labour:

    (i)   recumbent position – narrows outlet by inhibiting 'give' of pelvic joints and extension of coccyx

    (ii)   epidural analgesia – immobility and lack of pelvic floor tone leads to poor shoulder decent / rotation

Incidence:

Often quoted as 1–2% – depends on categorisation (Mortimore and McNabb 1998), i.e. are shoulders delayed or impacted?

Management (see Figure 12, p. 208):

Skill, judgement and the individual case dictate method / manoeuvre used, for example:

McRoberts manoeuvre:

With the mother in the dorsal position her knees are placed in an exaggerated knees–chest position; normal delivery of shoulders may now be possible

All-fours position

This can facilitate the delivery of the posterior shoulder first, which releases the trapped shoulder, enabling delivery.

Wood's or Rubin manoeuvres (usually by obstetrician)

These involve internal rotation of the fetal shoulders through 180 degrees.

Suprapubic pressure can be applied to release the trapped shoulder.

Zavanelli manoeuvre (by obstetrician)

Cephalic replacement followed by caesarean section

Complications:

Baby:

Perinatal mortality / morbidity

Birth asphyxia / hypoxia

Erb's palsy

Brachial plexus injury

Fractured clavicle or humerus – especially when traction used

Mother:

Uterine rupture – especially if fundal pressure used

Intrapartum or postpartum haemorrhage

Trauma – perineal; pelvic floor; cervical; haematoma formation

Long-term morbidity:

    (i)   physical

    (ii)   psychological

    (iii) social

    (iv) sexual

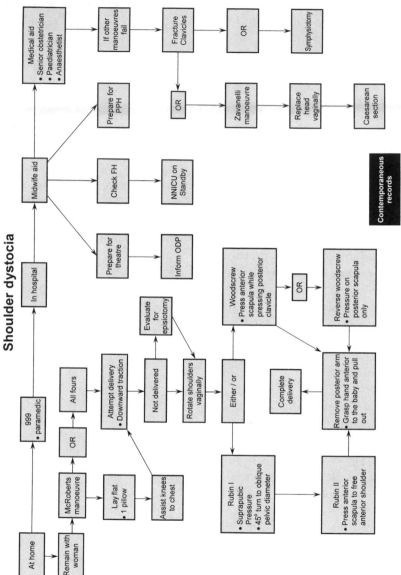

Figure 12 Shoulder dystocia

Student activity:

Note your local procedures

Further reading: Brunner *et al.* 1998; Guerewitsch *et al.* 2005; Nocon *et al.* 1993; Saunders 1997; Squire 2002

Sickle cell disease – see **haemoglobinopathies** in Section 2 above

Small for gestational age baby (SGA) (see also **pre-term baby** and **intrauterine growth retardation (IUGR)** in Section 2 above)

A baby below the 10th percentile for gestation, i.e. with IUGR (NB baby may also be pre-term); may be symmetrical or asymmetrical.

Characteristics:

	Asymmetrical	*Symmetrical*
(1) head	normal for gestation	small for gestation
	large for weight	normal for weight
	fontanelles normal	normal
	skull bones hard	skull bones hard
	eyes open	eyes open
(2) length	long for weight	normal for weight
(3) limbs	thin for size	normal for size
(4) muscle tone	normal	normal
(5) chest	ribs clearly visible	normal
	breast tissue normal	normal
(6) skin	loose, dry, scaling, cracked	normal
	nails long and firm	nails long and firm
	normal colour or meconium-stained	normal colour
	lack subcutaneous fat	lack subcutaneous fat
(7) abdomen	hollow	normal
	cord dries and separates early	thin cord separates early
(8) genitalia	normal	normal
(9) behaviour	alert and lively	alert
	very hungry	normal appetite
	eager to suck	normal sucking

Aetiology:

Asymmetrical growth retardation:

Occurs from third trimester – linked to diminished placental function due to:

    (i)   pre-eclampsia and hypertensive disorders

    (ii) smoking

    (iii) multiple pregnancy

    (iv) infarction after separation, e.g. APH, threatened abortion

Symmetrical growth retardation:

Develops early in pregnancy, e.g. due to:

  (often) no identifiable cause

  intrauterine infection

Maternal conditions:

    (i)   systemic / genital tract infections

    (ii)   blood disorders, e.g. anaemia; haemoglobinopathies

    (iii) chronic respiratory disease

    (iv) severe renal or cardiac disease

    (v)   metabolic disorders, e.g. PKU

    (vi) medications, e.g. steroids; cytotoxics; phenytoin (see **epilepsy** in Section 2 above)

    (vii) substance abuse, e.g. alcohol; drugs

    (viii) malnutrition

    (ix) low socio-economic status

Fetal conditions:

    (i)   inherited factors, e.g. small build; chromosomal abnormalities

    (ii) congenital abnormalities, e.g. cardiac; renal

    (iii) intrauterine infections, e.g. rubella and other viruses; toxoplasmosis

Management – initial

Delivery in consultant unit with NNICU (? *in utero* transfer – trained escort)

Paediatrician at delivery

Necessary resuscitation measures (see **birth asphyxia** in Section 2 above)

Thermoregulation (see **hypothermia – neonatal** in Section 2 above)

NNICU or transitional care prn

Weighed

Base-line observations:

    (i)   temperature

    (ii) respiratory rate – ? oxygen saturation

    (iii) heart rate

    (iv) blood glucose

Information and support to parents

Management – subsequent:

Depends on condition

Early feeding

? Blood glucose monitoring

? Infection screening

Thermoregulation

Monitor elimination

Hygiene and prevention of infection

Continue information and support for parents

Paediatric follow-up after discharge

Complications:

Symmetrically growth-retarded – poorer prognosis

Perinatal / neonatal mortality

Neurological damage from hypoxia (before, during, after birth)

Persistent fetal circulation

Increased risk of SIDS

Long-term physical / neurological morbidity, e.g. motor function / behaviour

Student activity:

Compare / contrast SGA / pre-term baby

Further reading: Curran *et al.* 1997

Smoking and pregnancy

Reasons women may smoke:

Aids coping with – anger; stress; frustration; poor home conditions

Peer pressure / fashion

Gives confidence

Physical / psychological dependence

Something to do / habit

Keep weight down

Give break / time for self

?Only purchase made for herself

Tobacco smoke:

Contains thousands of chemicals (metabolites found in urine, saliva, cervical secretions) – most dangerous being:

Carbon monoxide (CO):

Hb has a 200 times greater affinity for CO than O_2 (results in O_2 deficiency)

CO elimination from fetus slower than from mother

Increases blood viscosity (thick, sticky); leads to:

    (i)   increased thromboembolic disorders

    (ii) poorer circulation – poor O_2 perfusion – IUGR

    (iii) poor uterine circulation – IUGR

Nicotine:

Reaches brain 10 seconds after inhalation

Increases adrenaline / decreases noradrenaline – mood alteration:

(i)   lowers aggression / stress

(ii) increases tolerance

(iii) causes feeling of excitement

(iv) improves vigilance, concentration, speed / reaction time;

(v)   heightens arousal

(vi) lowers efficiency of food metabolism

(vii) lowers appetite

Aids release of catecholamines from adrenal and nerve cells, resulting in:

(i)   increase heart rate / vasoconstriction

(ii) increased O_2 consumption

(iii) increased use of free fatty acids – hypoglycaemia

(iv) lower placental blood flow / fetal breathing movements

Polycyclic aromatic hydrocarbons:

Interfere with normal enzyme transport

Hydrogen cyanide:

(i)   broken down into thiocyanate

(ii) lowers blood pressure (less risk of PIH)

(iii) lowers B_{12} levels

(iv) ? combines with amino acids – less protein available for fetal growth

Complications:

Short term:

Usually dose-related, i.e. number smoked daily / amount inhaled

? Link with passive smoking

Lowered fertility

Low oocyte production in assisted conception

?? Sperm damage

Spontaneous abortion rate considerably higher, more likely in 4th–7th month

Most harm to fetus after 4th month

Lower PIH, but more perinatal deaths if it does occur

Placenta praevia / abruption commoner

Low birth weight – approx. 170–200 g; lower if mother drinks alcohol

Increased perinatal mortality – cessation improves statistics

? Increased congenital abnormalities

Increased risk of PROM
Increased pre-term delivery
Increased fetal distress in labour; therefore operative / instrumental delivery
Lactation capacity down
Tobacco metabolites in breast milk
Early baby weaning commoner in smoking mothers

Long term:
Increased risk of:
SIDS
Infant mortality
Respiratory disease, e.g. bronchitis, pneumonia, asthma
Glue ear / hearing difficulty
Hospitalisation
Retarded physical / mental development
Vascular-related disease in later life
Leukaemia – twice the risk
Increase in all cancers
Twice as likely to smoke themselves

Management:
All smokers expect to be asked about smoking
Be non-judgemental – a dogmatic approach ? causes reluctance to attend
Elicit knowledge about smoking and pregnancy
Ask why she smokes
Ask how she feels about smoking – would like to stop / not

Not willing to stop:
Correct misinformation
Explain how smoking is harmful to the baby
Offer other information only if she wishes
Warn that likely to be asked again
Complete accurate records of discussion

Considering stopping / wishes to stop:
Correct misinformation
Explain how smoking is harmful to the baby
Explore potential difficulties in stopping
Elicit available family / friends support
Ask her what would help her to give up
Offer possible ideas to help, e.g.:

 (i) consider what it would be like not to smoke

 (ii) choose a day to stop

 (iii) dispose of remaining cigarettes, matches, lighter, ashtray

 (iv) make one room / whole house no smoking zone

 (v) ask for help from family / friends; they may join in!

 (vi) change routine to avoid usual smoking situations

 (vii) keep hands busy

 (viii) save the money towards baby clothes / equipment

Offer continued support yourself

Offer information about local / national support groups

Inform her that her progress will be questioned next visit

Complete accurate records of discussion

Student activity:

Review your local policy on smoking in pregnancy information-giving.

Find leaflets available in your unit.

Identify any local stop smoking support groups.

Further reading: Dimond 1996; Health Education Authority 1999; Lieberman *et al.* 1994; Lorente *et al.* 2000; Rantakallio *et al.* 1995; Thomson 1993a; Wisborg *et al.* 2001

Stillbirth – see **intrauterine death** in Section 2 above.

Stillbirth and Neonatal Death Society (SANDS)

A national charitable organisation based in London, with local branches and members, offering help and support to bereaved mothers and families following miscarriage, stillbirth or neonatal death. The society has highlighted the needs of bereaved parents and issued guidelines for service providers and practitioners on ways of improving services.

SANDS	Tel.	020 7436 5881 – helpline 10a.m.–3p.m.
23 Portland Place		Mon.–Fri.
London		020 7436 7940 – head office 10a.m.–5p.m.
W1B 1LY		Mon.–Fri.
	Fax.	020 7436 3715
	E-mail	support@uk-sands.org
	Web site	http://www.uk-sands.org

Strategic Health Authorities (SHAs)

The SHAs have the responsibility for strategic development and quality assurance in local NHS health services. They link Department of Health directives and national priorities with local service provison, e.g. improving cancer services and standards for the prevention of methicillin-resistant *Staphylococcus aureus* (MRSA) infection.

Substance-abusing mother and baby

Substances – (many abusers are poly (many) drug users):
  Alcohol
  Amphetamines, e.g. speed; ecstasy (E)
  Cocaine; crack cocaine
  Narcotics, e.g. heroin; morphine
  Cannabis
  Smoking (see separate category)
  Tranquillisers / sedatives, e.g. valium; temazepam
  Volatile liquids / gases

Methods of consumption:
  Ingestion, e.g. tablets; alcohol
  Inhalation, e.g. tobacco smoke; smoked heroin; vapours from glue / butane gas
  Transdermal, e.g. skin patches
  Rectally, e.g. ecstasy
  Snorting, e.g. cocaine
  IV, e.g. heroin; some non-IV substances, e.g. temazepam; methadone

Aetiology:
  Commonly multifactorial:
    Socio-economic / psychosocial factors
    Peer pressure
    Cultural influences
    Poor parenting
    Lack of education

Complications – general
  Poor nutrition
  Behavioural malfunction
  Criminal activity:
      (i)   prostitution (to pay for habit)
      (ii) sexual promiscuity
      (iii) violence
  Infections:
      (i)   general (poor resistance)
      (ii) STIs
      (iii) IV transmitted, e.g. hepatitis, HIV, septicaemia (shared equipment, non-aseptic technique)

Injury / death:
  (i)   accident
  (ii) overdose
  (iii) hyperpyrexia (ecstasy)
  (iv) inhaled vomit
Circulatory:
  (i)   thrombophlebitis
  (ii) abscess or fibrosis at IV site
  (iii) thrombo-embolism
  (iv) cardiac arrhythmias / arrest
Respiratory:
  (i)   nasal damage (cocaine)
  (ii) asthma / bronchitis
  (iii) respiratory arrest

Complications – maternal:

Amenorrhoea / infertility
Unrecognised / un-acknowledged pregnancy
Late / non-booking / poor attender antenatally
Absent family / friends support
Unable / unwilling to attend parent education
Poor knowledge about pregnancy, childbirth, parenting
Poor nutritional status, lack of vitamins, iron and folic acid
Pre-term labour

Complications – baby:

Spontaneous abortion
Chronic fetal hypoxia – IUGR
Fetal distress in labour / perinatal hypoxia
Pre-term birth / low birth weight
Perinatal death
Congenital abnormalities due to:
  (i) early intrauterine infection
  (ii) fetal alcohol syndrome
Neonatal thermoregulation difficulties
Neonatal drug addiction / withdrawal syndrome
Prolonged physical / mental morbidity

Management:

Pre-conception (ideally) to de-toxify / improve nutritional status
Antenatal:

(i)   early booking – non-judgemental approach

(ii)   thorough history – including substance(s) used (not always accurately given)

(iii) antenatal screening (esp. infection, e.g. hepatitis, HIV, STI prn)

(iv) nutritional advice

(v)   monitoring fetal well-being (diminished fetal breathing movements on USS)

(vi) referral / liaison – drug management team / midwife – ? methadone (liquid narcotic substitute) or buprenorphine (Subutex) (sublingual tablet) opiod replacement programme – slowly decreasing doses to lessen withdrawal symptoms / illicit drug use (sudden withdrawal ? fetal distress, abortion, pre-term labour)

(vii) encourage regular antenatal attendance, including parent education

(viii) liaison – social services / health visitor – ? attendance at case conference(s)

Labour:

(i)   continuous CTG

(ii)   pethidine ? ineffective – epidural suitable analgesia

(iii) paediatrician at delivery

(iv) no neonatal naloxone (Narcain) ? cause sudden withdrawal symptoms

(v)   ? neonatal unit on standby

Postnatal:

(i)   breast feeding ? suitable depending on individual circumstances (NB breast milk alcohol levels = maternal serum alcohol levels)

(ii)   continue liaison – multiprofessional team prn

(iii) additional support aids parenting skill development

(iv) continue methadone schedule

Neonate:

(i)   remains with mother if possible

(ii)   special care unit prn

(iii) possible withdrawal symptoms:

    (a) tremors, jitters, convulsions

    (b) diarrhoea

    (c) sneezing

    (d) high-pitched cry / very unsettled

    (e) sweating

    (f) feeding difficulties

    (iv) treat / manage withdrawal symptoms:
        (a) sedatives, anticonvulsants, ? morphine
        (b) prevent dehydration
        (c) comfort / soothing
    (v)   ? infection screening
    (vi) information / support mother
    (vii) ? long-term paediatric follow-up

Student activity:

Find out your local policy on management of mother / baby.

Sudden infant death syndrome (SIDS) (cot death)

The sudden death of an infant unexplained by history or post-mortem
  examination

Incidence:

309 in UK in 2004 – rate 0.43 per 1000 live births <12 months old (FSID
  2006)

75% fall in the rate since the Reduce the Risk campaign in England and Wales
  in 1991 (FSID 2006)

During 2000–2004 SIDS was responsible for 89% of all sudden deaths in
  England and Wales in babies < six months and is the leading cause of deaths
  in babies > one month of age (FSID 2006)

Aetiology:

Unclear – ? multifactorial, ? combined factors during a vulnerable time

Occurs any time from birth – incidence peaks at 2–3 months, but low incidence
  beyond 9 months

Risk factors:

Low birth weight (LBW)

Pre-term birth

Multiple birth

Male – higher incidence

Young maternal age – especially without supportive partner

High maternal parity – especially if <25 years

Short interval between pregnancies – <6 months

Low parental socio-economic status

Low parental educational achievement

Parental unemployment

Smoking – maternal smoking during pregnancy (Wisborg *et al.* 2001) (increases
  with number of cigarettes and with paternal smoking)

Infant passive smoking

Sleeping prone (on the front)

Overheating – excess bedding / clothing; room temperature; fever (NB temperature control mechanism inefficient); illness

Prevention:

Improved socio-economic factors, including family spacing

Ideally, prevent pre-term and LBW babies

Stop smoking before / during pregnancy; avoid baby passive smoking

Avoid overheating:

- (i) sleep supine (on back)
- (ii) room temperature 16°C–20°C
- (iii) head uncovered – baby's feet at cot bottom prevent slipping under bedding
- (iv) avoid direct heating – hot water bottle / radiant heat
- (v) no excess clothing, especially if unwell / fever
- (vi) ? no duvet (see Mitchell *et al.* 1999) or 'baby nests'

Monitor baby's general health / prompt medical attention prn

Parents taught CPR

Recent issues – unproven risks:

? Link dummy use / not

Caffeine consumption antenatally

Infant immunisation

Infants travelling by aeroplane

Toxic gases from mattresses

Student activity:

Note your local policies / available literature for parents.

Further reading: Bruce 1995; Carpenter *et al.* 2005; DoH 1996b; Fleming *et al.* 1999; Mitchell *et al.* 1999; Young and Fleming 1999.

For latest information http://www.sids.org.uk/fsid/

Symphysis pubis pain / sacro-iliac pain

Pain at / surrounding symphysis pubis joint, +/– sacro-iliac joint pain: increasingly diagnosed but still under-reported

Aetiology:

Pregnancy hormone link: i.e. progesterone and relaxin soften joint cartilage and relax supporting ligaments (pelvis 'gives' – more room for birth).

Occurs during pregnancy, labour, puerperium.

Joint inflammation, swelling; symphysis pubis diastasis (SPD) leads to joint movement.

Squatting position during pregnancy, labour, delivery strains joint

Unaccustomed exercise, especially involving leg abduction (opening out)

Large baby

CPD

Abnormal presentation

Precipitate labour

Difficult delivery

Careless leg abduction into lithotomy position (NB epidural may mask joint strain)

Signs and symptoms:

Joint / groin pain, ? radiates to thighs / lower back

Sensation of joint movement

Difficulty walking / weight-bearing, climbing stairs, getting into bed / bath

Waddling gait (walk)

Separation may be seen on X-ray / USS

Prevention:

Avoiding unaccustomed exercise / leg abduction (NB care in aquanatal exercises)

Avoid heavy lifting / use correct lifting technique

Abdominal support for woman with lax muscles

Correct management of labour, especially placing into lithotomy position

Management:

Depends on symptom severity

Bed rest, ? hospital, in most comfortable position – ? supported left lateral (NB – DVT prevention)

Obstetric physiotherapist referral

Pelvic binder – Tubigrip / Tubipad

Regular analgesia +/– anti-inflammatory drugs

Adduct legs (knees together) for movement between standing position and bed/chair

Minimise weight-bearing – wheelchair, elbow crutches, walking frame

Shower (use chair), not bath

Mobilisation as condition allows

Help / support at home

Consider labour / delivery position – have a 'dry run' – ? left lateral / 'all-fours'

Careful movement / lithotomy position when epidural, avoiding strain / worsening

Complications:

? Caesarean section if severe

Long-term social / psychological morbidity (chronic pain)

Talipes

A congenitally abnormal position of one / both feet

Aetiology:

Muscle and tendon contraction

? Genetic origin

Commonly from intrauterine position – breech, oligohydramnios (low liquor volume)

Recognition:

Part of midwife's initial neonatal examination

Management:

Depends on severity

Paediatric / physiotherapist referral

Passive exercises (teach mother)

Splinting

Surgery

Complications:

Delayed recognition prolongs treatment

Difficulty / inability walking

TAMBA – (Twins and Multiple Birth Association)

A national charity providing information to professionals and information and support to parents with twins or multiple pregnancy / births.

TAMBA	tel. 0870 770 3305 Mon.–Fri. 9.30–5.00 p.m.
2 The Willows	Fax. 0870 770 3303
Gardner Road,	http://www.tamba.org.uk/html/home.htm
Guildford, Surrey	
GU1 4PG	

Teenage pregnancy

Early teenage pregnancy = baby born to girl 16 years / younger

Has a major effect on physical, social, emotional well-being

UK has highest teenage pregnancy rate in Europe

Government initiatives developed to lower rate

Lack of sex education / knowledge may not be the reason for unplanned pregnancy – midwives are in a position to offer teenagers support, advice, referral to appropriate agencies

Specific parent education sessions may be provided for teenagers

Specific problems:

Delay in recognising pregnancy = late booking

Concealed pregnancy – no one to talk to

Late TOP – increased risks

Higher pregnancy complications:

      (i)   anaemia

      (ii)   PIH / pre-eclampsia / eclampsia

      (iii) APH

      (iv) pre-term birth / low birth weight babies / IUGR

      (v)   CPD

      (vi) fetal abnormalities / stillbirth

Socio-economic / psychological problems:

      (i)   high-risk activities – smoking, alcohol, drugs

      (ii)   poor nutrition

      (iii) poverty – especially <16 (unable to claim benefit themselves)

      (iv) rejection – family / partner

      (v)   incomplete education – affects long-term employment = poverty trap

      (vi) family stress / marital break-up / disputes over child care / rearing / domestic violence or abuse

Student activity:

Identify local initiatives to support / educate pregnant teenagers

Further reading: Bailey *et al.* 2004; DoH 2002; Hayes 2003; Kidger 2004; Nolan 1998; Shakespeare 2004; van den Akker *et al.* 1999

Temperature-taking

Aim:

Identification of pyrexia or hypothermia

Sites:

Oral – accurate

Rectal – accurate – higher reading than oral

Axilla – less accurate – lower reading than oral

Skin – ? accurate – much lower reading than oral

Ear (tympanic membrane) – accurate

Types of thermometer:
    Mercury-in-glass (normal / low reading) – oral, rectal, axilla
    Chemical / disposable – oral, axilla, skin – unsuitable for professional use
    Electronic – oral, skin, ear

Preparation:
    Explain procedure
    Ensure privacy prn
    Appropriate thermometer for site + disposable covers prn
    Ensure mercury in glass thermometer shaken down
    Gloves / lubricant for rectal
    Temperature chart

Action:
Oral:
    Unsuitable for neonate
    Apply disposable cover prn
    Gently insert bulb into posterior sublingual (under tongue) pocket
    Retained for minimum 2 min. (glass); 1 min. (chemical); until ready
        (electronic)
    Remove and read at eye level
    Clean / disinfect according to local policy
    Chart results

Axilla:
    Suitable for neonate
    Place thermometer in axilla centre
    Arm lowered and placed across chest
    Retained for 5 min. (glass); 3 min. (disposable); until ready (electronic)

Rectal:
    Unsuitable for neonate or those with rectal conditions
    Client turned on to side / knees bent
    With gloved hand, lubricate thermometer and gently insert into anus 3–4 cm
    Retain for 2 min.
    Remove, clean thermometer and anal area
    Return client to comfortable position
    Continue as above

Skin (electronic):
    Suitable for neonate
    Select appropriate site (abdomen common)

Fix with hypoallergenic tape
Connect to recording apparatus / incubator temperature control
Chart results

Tympanic:
Unsuitable for neonate
Apply disposable cover to thermometer speculum
Insert probe gently into ear canal
Reading within 1–2 seconds
Chart result

Student activity:
Note your local policies
Further reading: Severine and McKenzie 1999; Torrance and Semple 1998a,b

Tentorial tear
A torn tentorium cerebelli (a layer of the dura mater membrane between cerebrum and cerebellum)

Aetiology:
Sudden / excessive moulding of fetal skull during birth, because of e.g.:
- (i) OP position
- (ii) precipitate labour
- (iii) rapid second stage
- (iv) uncontrolled head of breech

Large / extended head
Prolonged labour
Operative delivery
Delicate skull – prematurity

Signs:
Birth asphyxia with slow / no recovery
Hypotonia (floppy), ? followed by hypertonia (stiff)
Signs of cerebral irritation:
- (i) irritability
- (ii) poor feeding
- (iii) lethargy
- (iv) vomiting
- (v) jittering / convulsions
- (vi) apnoea attack (stops breathing)
- (vii) shrill cry
- (viii) tense / bulging fontanelles

Management:
Paediatrician
NNICU
Gentle handling
Monitor vital signs
Stabilisation of blood gases and glucose, temperature
Control convulsions
IV fluids
Konakion (vitamin K_1) 0.5 mg or 1.0 mg IV / IM
Paediatric follow-up

Consequences:
Concurrent tearing of large vein (vein of Galen)
Cerebral haemorrhage
Neonatal death
Neurological damage
Long-term morbidity

Term Breech Trial

A multicentre, international randomised controlled trial of planned caesarean section vs. planned vaginal delivery of the breech fetus at term, to identify the best approach to management. Began in January 1997, ending in July 2000. Centres included Argentina, Canada, Chile, Finland, India, UK and USA, with Canada funding and coordinating the project.

Inclusion criteria included: pregnancy minimum of 37 weeks; frank (extended) or flexed (not footling) breech presentation; live fetus; no evidence of CPD. Exclusion criteria included estimated fetal size 4000 g or more and contraindications to vaginal delivery.

Results indicated that caesarean section to deliver the breech at term resulted in lower perinatal mortality and morbidity and no increase in serious maternal consequences.

Student activity:
Further reading: Hannah *et al.* 2000

Thalassaemia – see **haemoglobinopathies** in Section 2 above

Transverse / oblique lie

Non-longitudinal lie of the fetus with shoulder presentation

Aetiology:
>   Lax uterine / abdominal muscles (grand(e) multiparity)
>   Placenta praevia
>   Polyhydramnios
>   Multiple pregnancy
>   Abnormal uterus
>   Uterine fibroid
>   Abnormal pelvis

Diagnosis:
>   Abdominal palpation:
>   >   (i)   fundus is low / abdomen broad
>   >   (ii) head is felt laterally
>   Ultrasound scan

Management:
>   >32–34 weeks obstetric referral
>   USS – identify cause / exclude abnormalities
>   >37 weeks ? ECV
>   Inform woman urgent admission if SRM
>   At term ? ECV and immediate induction of labour with Syntocinon
>   ? ARM (senior obstetrician) once head enters pelvis
>   Continuous electronic monitoring in labour
>   Emergency caesarean section prn

Complications:
>   Obstructed labour
>   Cord prolapse

Twins – see **multiple pregnancy** in Section 2 above

Urinary tract infection – UTI (see also **cystitis** in Section 2 above)
Bacterial infection of the urinary tract (bladder = cystitis, kidney = nephritis or
    pyelonephritis), commonly by *E.coli* (normal bowel flora)

Aetiology in pregnancy:
>   Relaxation of smooth muscle of the ureters due to progesterone causes
>   urinary stasis
>   Short female urethra compounded by poor hygiene increases ascending
>   organisms

Aetiology in neonate:

Susceptibility to transmission of organisms, especially if low birth weight

Signs and symptoms (adult):	*Signs and symptoms (neonate):*
general malaise (feeling unwell)	jaundice
vomiting	vomiting
pyrexia	normal / unstable temperature
abdominal / loin pain or tenderness	diarrhoea
frequency of micturition – ? painful	
offensive urine	
haematuria (blood in urine)	
uterine contractions possible	

Management:

History

General observations – condition, temperature, pulse

MSSU

High fluid intake – oral / IVI

Appropriate antibiotics (see **ORACLE trial** related to the prevention of pre-term labour)

Uterine relaxants if danger of pre-term labour

Treat neonatal jaundice

Uterine inversion

A uterus partially / completely inside out – fundus above the cervix / protruding at vulva

Aetiology:

Spontaneous – precipitate labour / poor uterine tone

Third- stage mismanagement – excess fundal pressure / cord traction as uterus relaxed

Short cord – pulls fundus down during the birth

Manual removal of placenta – continued fundal pressure as the hand is removed from the uterus

Signs and symptoms:

Fundus visualised at vagina / felt on VE

Severe pain

Excessive bleeding / PPH

No uterus palpated abdominally

Shock – neurological (nerve / ligament traction) and /or haemorrhagic

Management – initial (see Figure 13, p. 229):
Replace the uterus manually – hydrostatic pressure may help
Do not attempt to remove placenta

Management – subsequent:
Encourage postnatal exercises
Debriefing

Complications:
Profound shock – renal damage; Sheehan's syndrome
Sepsis
Psychological trauma
Anxiety in subsequent pregnancies

Student activity:
Note local policies. Further reading: Kroll and Lyne 2002

Uterine rupture
Complete:
Perforation of the myometrium and perimetrium, with the fetus expelled through
the uterine wall; placenta separates.

Incomplete:
The perimetrium remains intact containing the fetus, and may stop the placenta
from separating.

Aetiology:
Cause unclear
One or a combination of:
- (i) prostaglandin / oxytocic misuse
- (ii) weak scar tissue – previous surgery, e.g. caesarean section / uterine evacuation
- (iii) instrumental delivery – especially using Kielland's forceps
- (iv) extended cervical tear
- (v) severe placental abruption
- (vi) intrauterine manipulation, e.g. in shoulder presentation
- (vii) placenta accreta (i.e. morbidity adhered to uterus)

Signs and symptoms:
Often dramatic in complete – possibly 'silent' in incomplete
Severe constant abdominal pain

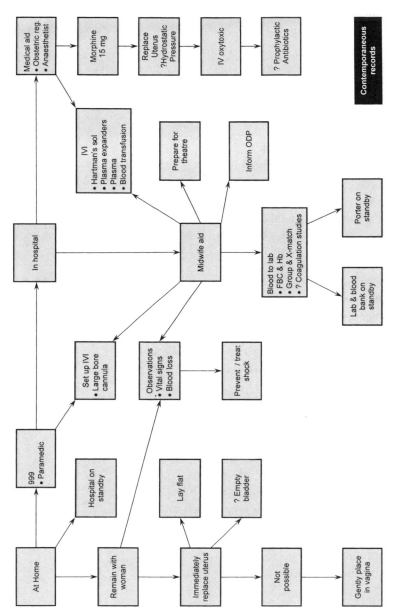

Figure 13 Uterine inversion

Tender uterine scar
Reduced contractions
Vaginal bleeding
Tachycardia
Hypotension, shock and collapse
Fetal distress
IUD
Fetal parts felt outside uterus
Seen at caesarean section

Prevention:
Woman with uterine scar:
Senior obstetrician-led care (antenatal / intrapartum)
Hospital birth in a consultant unit
Avoid / cautious use of prostaglandins / oxytocics
Close intrapartum fetal / maternal monitoring
Early referral to senior obstetrician if symptomatic

General:
Appropriately used / managed prostaglandins / oxytocics (close fetal / maternal monitoring – avoid complacency)
Senior obstetrician for Kielland's forceps / intrauterine manipulation – ? caesarean section
Forceps delivery only when cervix fully dilated
Avoid maternal pushing when cervix not fully dilated

Management:
Initial (see Figure 14, p. 231):

Subsequent:
Close monitoring – ? special / intensive care
Debriefing
Bereavement care if perinatal death
Psychological support – especially if hysterectomy
Consider future pregnancies, e.g. timing, management

Complications:
Severe haemorrhage
DIC
Maternal death
    5 between 1994–1996 (Lewis 1998)
    1 between 1997–1999 (Lewis 2001)
    1 between 2000–2002 (Lewis 2004)

Uterine rupture

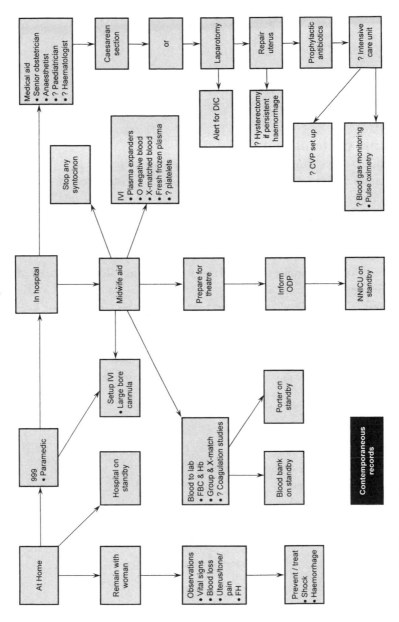

Figure 14 Uterine rupture

Perinatal death
Complicated subsequent pregnancies
Hysterectomy / infertility
Long-term psychological problems

Student activity:
Note your local policy.
Familiarise yourself with local intensive care charts/records.
Further reading: Kroll and Lyne 2002; Saunders 1997

Vaginal examination (VE)
An intimate procedure that is part of the midwife's role
May cause distress, discomfort, embarrassment – consider the possible response
of survivors of sexual abuse

Indications:
Confirm labour onset / assess progress
Assess state of membranes / perform ARM (see **artificial rupture of membranes** in Section 2 above)
Assess fetal position / presentation
Exclude / diagnose cord prolapse in SRM
Apply fetal scalp electrode (FSE)
Confirm full cervical dilatation, i.e. second-stage labour
Identify second twin's presenting part / ARM second amniotic sac

Aim:
Accurate assessment
Minimise infection risk
Maintain woman's dignity / inform of findings
Keep accurate records

Preparation:
Trolley – VE pack, cleansing solution, obstetric cream, sterile gloves, ?
Amnihook
Partogram to record findings
Note timing last VE (commonly 4-hourly)
Explain procedure / seek consent
Ensure privacy
Woman empties bladder
Perform abdominal palpation

Action:

Woman in dorsal position, knees bent, thighs abducted, relaxed

Aseptic technique – gloves worn

Vulva swabbed using left hand (thus avoiding contamination) – note external genitalia

Two fingers of right hand inserted gently using lubrication

Assess vaginal condition – ? warm / moist

Feel cervix – consistency ? soft / firm; length ? effaced / not; dilatation; application to presenting part

Feel for forewaters – ? present / absent / bulging – following ARM exclude cord prolapse

Confirm level of presenting part, i.e. station in relation to pelvic landmarks

Feel for landmarks on fetal skull – determines position

Note caput formation / moulding

Assess ischial spines – ? prominent; angle of pubic arch

Remove fingers – note show / liquor

Make woman comfortable / explain findings

Record information accurately

Medical aid prn

Student activity:

Note local policies and procedures

Further reading: Hobbs 2003; Stuart 2003; Warren 2003

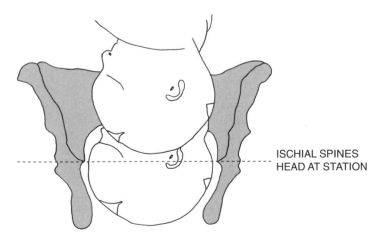

ISCHIAL SPINES
HEAD AT STATION

Diagram 6 Stations of the head in the pelvis

Varicose veins (see also **haemorrhoids** in Section 2 above)
Enlarged veins commonly in:
Lower leg

Vulva

Anal / rectal area (haemorrhoids)

Pelvic veins

Aetiology:
Weakened valves +/or vein walls – poor venous return

Common antenatally – increased venous stasis caused by:

      (i)   gravid uterus raising abdominal pressure

     (ii)   large baby

    (iii) multiple pregnancy

    (iv) polyhydramnios

     (v)   progesterone relaxing smooth muscle of veins

Signs and symptoms:
Visible superficially as dark blue lines / bulges

Deep leg / rectal veins not visible

Aching / heavy sensation

Oedema

Local inflammation

Pain / blood on passing stool (haemorrhoids)

Prevention / management:
Avoid prolonged standing

Elevate legs / pelvis (NB supine hypotension)

Legs:
Support tights / TED stockings (see terms) to prevent DVT (see Section 1 above)

Vulva:
Thick cotton sanitary pad for support

Care at delivery

Haemorrhoids:
Avoid constipation with high-fibre diet, adequate fluid intake, mild laxative, e.g. Lactulose

Complications:
Increased risk of thrombophlebitis / DVT

Pain / discomfort

Ruptured vulval veins / haemorrhage at delivery
Irritation / bleeding haemorrhoids
Long-term morbidity – pain / aching, stress about appearance

Venepuncture

Aim: obtain specimen of venous blood for laboratory tests

Preparation:

Tray with:

Appropriate colour-coded, correctly labelled vacutainer / similar or blood bottles, needle and syringe

Skin-cleansing swab

Tourniquet

? Gloves – personal preference (NB health and safety)

Skin plaster / micropore tape

Sterile cotton wool / gauze swabs

Laboratory request forms

Sharps container

Action:

Identify client / explain procedure / seek consent

Client sitting comfortably

Elicit which arm preferred

Inspect / determine which vein suitable – commonly median basilic (at elbow)

Apply tourniquet on upper arm

Prepare containers / needle and syringe

Cleanse area with swab

Insert needle into vein at angle of 15°

Obtain specimen(s) label tubes with client's personal details:

(i)   tubes without additives first

(ii) then coagulation tubes

(iii) finally tubes with additives prn

Release tourniquet

Remove needle / apply pressure with dry cotton wool

Apply plaster / gauze and micropore tape

Dispose of equipment safely

Dispatch to laboratory

Record in case notes

Student activity:

Note your unit policy for venepuncture, training required

Further reading: Campbell 1995

Ventouse delivery – see **instrumental delivery** in Section 2 above

Vomiting – see **nausea and vomiting** in Section 2 above

Winterton Report (1992) Parlimentary Select Committee on Health.
Second report on the maternity services
A major report published by the Health Committee of the House of Commons:
chair Nicholas Winterton. After a year-long enquiry collecting evidence from
mothers and midwives in Sweden, the Netherlands, Belfast, Cardiff, Leeds,
Oxford and elsewhere, the report gave recommendations to improve maternity
services. Some have been implemented: e.g. that women should be partners in
their more community-based care, greater professional continuity, promotion
of breast feeding, a paramedic service able to deal with obstetric emergencies,
and client-held notes. Others, e.g. raising maternity benefits for the young and
low-paid, improvement in status, pay and conditions for midwives, and trainee
status for SHOs under midwives' supervision, have not been accepted.
The report led to the setting up of an Expert Maternity Group under Baroness
Cumberlege, which resulted in the publication of *Changing Childbirth* by the
Department of Health in 1993.

References

Albers, L. L. (2000) Health problems after childbirth. *Journal of Midwifery and Women's Health* 45(1) January/February: 55–7

Albrechtsen, S., Rasmussen, S., Reigstad, H., *et al.* (1997) Evaluation of a protocol for selecting fetuses in breech presentation for vaginal delivery or caesarean section. *American Journal of Obstetrics and Gynaecology* September. 177 (3): 586–92 Abstract in: *MIDIRS Midwifery Digest* June 1998. 8 (2): 213

Almond, P. (1996) How health visitors assess the health of postnatal women. *Health Visitor* December. 69 (12): 495–8

Annapoora, V., Arulkumaran, S., Anandakumar, C., *et al.* (1997) External cephalic version at term with tocolysis and vibroacoustic stimulation. *International Journal of Gynaecology and Obstetrics* October. 59 (1): 13–18

APEC (1994) *Fact Sheet 1: Low-Dose Aspirin forHigh-Risk Pregnancy.* Action on Pre-eclampsia (registered charity), Abbots Langley, Herts

Arulkumaran, S. and Symonds, I. M. (1999) Psychosocial support or active management of labour or both to improve the outcome of labour. *British Journal of Obstetric and Gynaecology* July. 106 (7): 617–19

Bailey, N., Brown, G., Di Marco, H., *et al.* (2004) Teenage pregnancy: medical encounters. *British Journal of Midwifery* Nov. 12 (11): 680–5

Baker, C. (1996) Nutrition and hydration in labour *British Journal of Midwifery* November. 4 (11): 568–72

Barwise, C. (1998) Episiotomy and decision making. *British Journal of Midwifery* December. 6 (12): 787–90

Baston, H. (2004) Perineal repair. *Practising Midwife* Oct. 7 (9): 12–15

Bennet, V. R. and Brown, L. K. (2003) Chapter 7: The female pelvis and reproductive organs. In *Myles Textbook for Midwives* 14th edition (eds D. M. Fraser and M. A. Cooper). Churchill Livingstone, Edinburgh

Bennett, P. (1994) Pre-eclampsia I: the midwife and detection. *Modern Midwife* October: 20–2

Berry, H. (1997) Feast or famine? Oral intake during labour: current evidence and practice. *British Journal of Midwifery* July. 5 (7): 413–17

Bharj, K. (1995) Providing midwifery care in a multi-cultural society. *British Journal of Midwifery* May. 3 (5): 271–2, 274–7

Bick, D. (1999) The benefits of breastfeeding for the infant. *British Journal of Midwifery* May. 7 (5): 312–19

Bott, J. (1999a) Reflections on postnatal depression. *British Journal of Midwifery* January. 7 (1): 45–8

Bott, J. (1999b) HIV risk reduction and the use of universal precautions. *British Journal of Midwifery* November. 7 (11): 671–5

Bott, J. (2000a) HIV Screening issues for midwives. *British Journal of Midwifery* 8 (2): 72–8

Bott, J. (2000b) HIV and women: health and childbearing issues. *British Journal of Midwifery* January. 8 (1): 15–19

Boulvain, M., Stan, C. and Irion, O. (2005) Membrane sweeping for induction of labour. *The Cochrane Database of Systemic Reviews* Issue 1. Art. No. CD000451. DOI: 10.1002/14651858.CD000451.pub2

Boyle, M. (2002) *Emergencies Around Childbirth*. Radcliffe Medical Press, Abingdon, Oxon.

Briscoe, L., Clark, S. and Yoxall, C. W. (2002) Can transcutaneous billirubinometry reduce the need for blood tests in jaundiced full term babies? *Archives of Diseases of Childhood. Fetal and Neonatal Edition* May. 83 (3) F190–2

Bruce, M. (1995) Teaching parents CPR skills: parental confidence and a neonatal resuscitation programme. *Journal of Neonatal Nursing* 1 (3): 27–30

Brunner, J. P., Drummond, S. B., Meenan, A. L., *et al.* (1998) All-fours manoeuvre for reducing shoulder dystocia during labour. *Journal of Reproductive Medicine* May. 43 (5): 39–43 Reprinted in *MIDIRS Midwifery Digest* 1998, Dec. 8 (4): 466–8

Campbell, J. (1995) Making sense of the technique of venepuncture. *Nursing Times* 2nd August. 91 (31): 29–31

Carpenter, R. G., Waite, A., Coombs, R. C., *et al.* (2005) Repeat sudden unexpected and unexplained infant deaths: natural or unnatural? *The Lancet* 365 (9453): 29–35

Casson, I. F., Clarke, C. A., Howard, C. V., *et al.* (1997) Outcomes of pregnancy in insulin dependent diabetic women: results of a five year population cohort study. *British Medical Journal* 2nd August. 315: 275–8

CESDI (1999) *6th Annual Report*. Maternal and Child Health Research Consortium, London

Chan, J. Y. K. (1995) Dietary beliefs of Chinese patients. *Nursing Standard* 29th March. 9 (27): 30–4

Chappell, L. C., Seed, P. T., Briley, A. N., *et al.* (1999) Effect of antioxidants on the occurrence of pre-eclampsia in women at increased risk: a randomised trial. *The Lancet* 4th September. 354 (9181): 810–16

Chesney, M. (1995) The importance of cultural beliefs. *British Journal of Midwifery* May. 3 (5): 268–71

Cheung, F. (1996a) Background and cosmology of Chinese diet therapy in childbearing. *Midwives* June. 109 (1301): 146–9

Cheung, F. (1996b) Diet therapy in the postnatal period from a Chinese perspective. *Midwives* July. 109 (1301): 190–3

Clarkson, L. J. (2001) Retinopathy of prematurity: Part 1 A fresh look at its cause. *Journal of Neonatal Nursing* 7 (6): 186–9

Clarkson, L. J. (2002) Retinopathy of prematurity: Part 2. Current treatment options. *Journal of Neonatal Nursing* 8 (1): 7–10

Clements, S. and Reed, B. (1999) To stitch or not to stitch? A long term follow-up study of women with unsutured perineal tears. *The Practising Midwife* April. 2 (4): 20–8

Cluett, E. R., Alexander, J. and Pickering, R. M. (1995) Is measuring postnatal symphysis–fundal distance worthwhile? *Midwifery* 11 (4): 174–83

Coates, T. (2003) Chapter 30: Malpositions of the occiput and malpresentations. In *Myles Textbook for Midwives* 14th edition (eds D. M. Fraser and M. A. Cooper). Churchill Livingstone, Edinburgh

Coombes, J. (2000) Cholestasis in pregnancy: a challenging disorder. *British Journal of Midwifery* 8 (9): 565–70

Cornwell, S. and Dale, A. (1995) Lavender oil and perineal repair. *Modern Midwife* March: 31–3

Cowan, T. (1997) Blood glucose monitoring. *Professional Nurse* May. 2 (8): 593, 595–7

Crafter, H. (2002) Chapter 10: Intrapartum and primary post partum haemorrhage. In *Emergencies Around Childbirth: A Handbook for Midwives* (ed. M. Boyle). Radcliffe Medical Press, Abingdon, Oxon.

Crompton, J. (1996) Post-traumatic stress disorder and childbirth: 2. *British Journal of Midwifery* July. 4 (7): 354–6, 373

Curran, A., Brighton, J. and Murphy, V. (1997) Psychological care of parents of children in a NNICU and results of a questionnaire. *Journal of Neonatal Nursing* 3 (1): 25–9

Currid, T. (2004) Clinical issues relating to puerperal psychosis and its management. *Nursing Times* 27 Apr. 100 (17): 40–3

Davies, B. R. (2003) Early detection and treatment of postnatal depression in primary care. *Journal of Advanced Nursing* 44 (3): 248–55

Davis, A. (1998) Chlamydia: the most common sexually transmitted infection. *Nursing Times* 4th February. 94 (5) 56–8

Dimond, B. (1996) Smoking mothers' rights and the maternity unit. *Modern Midwife*. June: 10–11

Dimond, B. (1997) CESDI 2: the legal implications. *Modern Midwife* December: 7 (12): 20–2

Dimond, B. (1998) Complementary medicine in midwifery. *The Practising Midwife* April. 1 (4): 12–13

Dimond, B. (2000) The duty of quality and midwifery services. *British Journal of Midwifery* January. 8 (1): 20–3

Dimond, B. (2002) *Legal Aspects of Midwifery*. Books for Midwives, Edinburgh

DoH (Department of Health) (1993) *Changing Childbirth. Report of the Expert Maternity Group*. HMSO, London

DoH (Department of Health) (1996a) *Breastfeeding: Good Practice Guide to the NHS*. Department of Health, London

DoH (Department of Health) (1996b) *Confidential Enquiry into Stillbirths and Deaths in Infancy. Third Annual Report.* Executive summary and recommendations concentrating on the first two years of combined studies on sudden unexpected deaths in infancy. HMSO, London

DoH (Department of Health) (1997) *The New NHS – Modern, Dependable.* Department of Health, London

DoH (Department of Health) (1998) *Vitamin K for Newborn Babies.* 5 May. Department of Health, London. Reprinted in *MIDIRS Midwifery Digest* September. 8 (3): 350

DoH (Department of Health) (2002) Government response to the first annual report of the Independent Advisory Group on Teenage Pregnancy. http:// www.gov.uk

Draycott, T., Broad, G. and Chidley, K. (2000) The development of an eclampsia box and 'fire drill'. *British Journal of Midwifery* January. 8 (1): 26–30

Duley, L. (1995) Which anticonvulsant for women with eclampsia? Evidence from the Collaborative Eclampsia Trial. *The Lancet* 10th June. 345: 1455–63

Duley, L. and Watkins, K. (1999) The magpie trial: magnesium sulphate for pre-eclampsia. *British Journal of Midwifery* October. 7 (10): 617–19

Duley, L., Gülmezoglu, A. M. and Henderson-Smart, D. J. (2003) Magnesium sulphate and other anticonvulsants for women with pre-eclampsia. *The Cochrane Database of Systematic Reviews* Issue 2. Art. No. CD 000025. DOI: 10.1002/14651858.CD000025

Dyke, R. (1998) Surveying midwives' knowledge of toxoplasmosis. *RCM Midwives Journal.* May. 1 (5): 144–7

Edwards, G., Gordon, U. and Atherton, J. (2005) Network approach boosts midwives' public health role. *British Journal of Midwifery* January. 13 (1): 48–53

Ellwood, J. L. (1999) Survey of obstetricians understanding of the phrase '37 completed weeks' in the definition of term. *British Journal of Obstetrics and Gynaecology* September. 106 (9): 1000

Emery, M. L. (2000) Antenatal assessment of fetal well-being: neonatal consequences. *Journal of Neonatal Nursing* 6 (4): 123–6

Every, M. (1994) Meeting Report: CLASP trial. *Midwives Chronicle and Nursing Notes* October. 107 (1281): 402

Finigan, V. and Davies, S. (2004) 'I just wanted to love, hold him forever': women's lived experience of skin-to-skin contact with their baby immediately after birth. *Evidence Based Midwifery* 2 (2): 59–65

Fleming, P. J., Blair, P. S., Pollard, K., *et al.* (1999) Pacifier use and sudden infant death syndrome: results from the CESDI / SUDI case control study. *Archives of Diseases in Childhood.* August. 81 (2): 112–16

Foster, A. (1996) Perinatal bereavement support for families and midwives. *Midwives.* August. 109 (1303): 218–19

Fraser, D. M. and Cooper, M. A. (2003) *Myles Textbook for Midwives* 14th edition. Churchill Livingstone, Edinburgh

FSID (2006) Cot death facts and figures. Foundation for the Study of Infant Deaths. www.sids.org.uk/fsid/facts.htm (accessed 24/2/2006)

Gardosi, J. and Francis, A. (1999) Controlled trial of fundal height measurement plotted on customised antenatal growth charts. *British Journal of Obstetrics and Gynaecology* 106: 309–17

Gaskell, C. (1999) A review of puerperal psychosis. *British Journal of Midwifery* March. 7 (3): 172–4

Gemynthe, A., Langhoff-Ross, J., Sahl, S. and Knudsen, J. (1996) New Vicryl™ formulation: an improved method of perineal repair? *British Journal of Midwifery* May. 4 (5): 230–4

Gibbon, K. (2004) Developments in perinatal mental health assessments. *British Journal of Midwifery* December. 12 (12): 754–60

Greenough, A. (1997) Hope for infants with respiratory distress syndrome. Replacement surfactant therapy. *Professional Care of Mother and Child* 7 (4): 99–100

Greer, P. (1998) Vaginal thrush: diagnosis and treatment options. *Nursing Times* 28th January. 94 (4): 50–2

Gregorie, A. (1995) Hormones and postnatal depression. *British Journal of Midwifery* 3rd February. (2): 99–103

Guerewitsch, E. D., Kim, E. J., Yang, J. H., *et al.* (2005) Comparing McRobert's and Rubin's maneuvers for initial managment of shoulder dystocia: an objective evaluation. *American Journal of Obstetric and Gynecology* January. 192 (1): 153–60

Hamilton, A. (2003) Chapter 31: Operative delivery. In *Myles Textbook for Midwives* 14th edition (eds D. M. Fraser and M. A. Cooper). Churchill Livingstone, Edinburgh

Hannah, M. E., Hannah, W. J. and Hewson, S. A. (2000) Planned caesarean section versus planned vaginal birth for breech presentation at term: a randomised multicentre trial. *The Lancet* 21st October. 356: 1375–83

Harden, A. (1999) Sixteen to nineteen year olds' use of, and beliefs about, contraceptive services. *The British Journal of Family Planning* 24: 141–4

Hart, S. C. (1999) So what exactly is clinical governance? *British Journal of Midwifery* March. 7 (3): 175

Hayes, L. (2003) PN plus. 13b: teenage pregnancy – prevention and intervention *Practice Nurse* 28th Nov. 26 (9): 63–7

HEA (Health Education Authority) (1999) *Action on Smoking and Pregnancy: Information Pack*. Health Education Authority, London

Henderson, J. J., Evans, S. F., Straton, J. A. Y., *et al.* (2003) Impact of postnatal depression on breastfeeding duration. *Birth* September. 30 (3): 175–80

Hendrick, V. (2003) Treatment of postnatal depression: effective interventions are available, but the condition remains underdiagnosed. *British Medical Journal* 1st November. 327 (7422): 1003–4

Hennings, J., Williams, J. and Haque, B. N. (1996) Exploring the health needs of Bangladeshi women: a case study in using qualitative research methods. *Health Education Journal* 55: 11–23

Herbst, A. and Ingemarsson, I. (1994) Intermittent versus continuous electronic monitoring in labour: a randomised study. *British Journal of Obstetrics and Gynaecology*. August. 101: 663–8

Hibbard, B. M. *et al.* (1994) *Report on the Confidential Enquiry into Maternal Deaths in UK 1988–90*. HMSO, London

Hibbard, B. M. *et al.* (1996) *Report on the Confidential Enquiry into Maternal Deaths in UK 1991–93*. HMSO, London

Hobbs, L. (2003) Assessing cervical dilatation without VEs: watching the purple line. In *Midwifery Best Practice* (ed. S. Wickham). Books for Midwives Press, Edinburgh

Hodgson, T. (1994) Aromatherapy – a note of caution for midwives. *Modern Midwife* January: 31–3

Jones, E. (1995) Strategies to promote pre-term breastfeeding. *Modern Midwife* March: 8–11

Jones, K. (1999) Relief of heartburn and constipation during pregnancy. *British Journal of Midwifery* April. 7 (4): 228–30

Karpatkin, M. (1999) Coagulation problems in the newborn. *Semin. Neonatal* (4): 67–73

Kelly, M. E. (1999) Family planning: a consideration of the issues. *British Journal of Midwifery* Feb. 7 (2): 102–6

Kennedy, H. P. and MacDonald, E. L. (2002) 'Altered consciousness' during childbirth: potential clues to post traumatic stress disorder? *Journal of Midwifery and Women's Health* September/October. 47 (5): 380–2

Kenyon, S. (1995) ORACLE – an overview of the evidence. *MIDIRS Midwifery Digest* March. 5 (1): 14–16

Kenyon, S., Boulvain, M. and Neilson, J. (2004) Antibiotics for preterm rupture of the membranes: a systematic review. *Obstetrics Gynecology* November. 104(5 part 1): 1051–7

Kenyon, S. and Taylor, D. J. (2002) The effects of the publication of a major clinical trial in a high impact journal on clinical practice: the ORACLE trial experience *British Journal of Obstetrics and Gynaecology* 109 (12): 1341–3

Kidger, J. (2004) Including young mothers: limitations to New Labour's strategy for supporting teenage parents. *Critical Social Policy* August. 24 (3): 291–311

Kimber, L. (1998) Effective techniques for massage in labour. *The Practising Midwife* April. 1 (4): 36–9

King, J. and Flenady, V. (2002) Prophylactic antibiotics for inhibiting preterm labour with intact membranes. *The Cochrane Database of Systemic Reviews* 2002 Issue 4 Accessed 15/02/05

Kirsten, L., Dardeno, M. D. and Burkman, T. (1999) The intrauterine contraceptive device: an often-forgotten and maligned method of contraception. *American Journal of Obstetrics and Gynaecology* July. 181 (1): 1–5

Kroll, D. and Lyne, M. (2002) Chapter 8: Uterine inversion and uterine rupture. In *Emergencies Around Childbirth: A Handbook for Midwives* (ed. M. Boyle). Radcliffe Medical Press, Abingdon, Oxon

Kumar, R., Marks, M. and Jackson, K. (1995) Prevention and treatment of postnatal psychiatric disorders. *British Journal of Midwifery*. June. 3 (6): 314–17

Laing, K. G. (2001) Post-traumatic stress disorder: myth or reality? *British Journal of Midwifery* 9 (7): 447–52

Lang, S. (1994) Cup-feeding: an alternative method. *Midwives Chronicle and Nursing Notes*. May. 107 (1276): 171–6

Lavin, J. and Smith, A. R. B. (1996) Pelvic floor damage. *Modern Midwife*. May: 14–16

Layton, S. (2004) The effects of perineal trauma on women's health. *British Journal of Midwifery* 12 April (4): 231–6

Lee, B. (2002) Are you sitting comfortably? Issues around perineal trauma. *RCM Midwives Journal* September. 5 (9): 298–301

Lewis, G. (ed.) (1998) *Why Mothers Die. 1994–1996. Report on the Confidential Enquiries into Maternal Deaths in the United Kingdom.* HMSO, London

Lewis, G. (ed.) (2001) *Why Mothers Die 1997–1999. Report on the Confidential Enquiries into Maternal Deaths in the United Kingdom.* RCOG Press, London

Lewis, G. (ed.) (2004) *Why Mothers Die 2000–2004. Confidential Enquiry into Maternal and Child Health.* RCOG Press, London

Libbus, M. K. (2001) Review: oral and intravaginal agents are equally effective for treatment of uncomplicated vulvovaginal candidiasis. *Evidence Based Nursing* Oct. 4 (4): 112

Lieberman, E., Gremy, I., Lang, J. M. and Cohen, A. P. (1994) Low birth weight at term and the timing of fetal exposure to maternal smoking. *American Journal of Public Health* 84 (7): 1127–31

Lindqvist, A., Norden-Lindeberg, S. and Hanson, U. (1997) Perinatal mortality and route of delivery in term breech presentations. *British Journal of Obstetrics and Gynaecology* November. 104 (11): 1288–91 Abstract in: *MIDIRS Midwifery Digest* March 1998. 8 (1): 77

Lorente, C., Cordier, S., Goujard J., *et al.* (2000) Tobacco and alcohol use during pregnancy and risk of oral clefts. *American Journal of Public Health* 90 (3): 415–19

Lyons, C. M. (1995) Child protection and the Civil Law. In *The Child Protection Handbook* (eds K. Wilson and A. James). Baillière Tindall, London

McCandlish, R. (1999) The HOOP study: a personal view. *MIDIRS Midwifery Digest* March. 9 (1): 77–8

McCandlish, R. *et al.* (1998) A randomised controlled trial of care of the perineum during second stage of normal labour. *British Journal of Obstetrics and Gynaecology* December. 105 (12): 1262–72. Abstract in *MIDIRS Midwifery Digest* March 1999. 9 (1): 76

McDermott, E. (2001) Much ado about nothing? Diagnosis and management of obstetric cholestasis. *The Practising Midwife* 4 (4): 14–17

McDonald, S. (2002) Chapter 4: Pre-eclampsia and eclampsia. In *Emergencies Around Childbirth: A Handbook for Midwives* (ed. M. Boyle). Radcliffe Medical Press, Abingdon, Oxon

Machover, I. (1995) Turn, baby, turn! *Midwives* November. 108 (1294): 389–91

Mantle, F. (2001) The role of alternative medicine in treating postnatal depression. *British Journal of Community Nursing* 6 (7): 363–8

Marchant, S., Alexander, J. and Garcia, J. (2000) How does it feel to you? *Practising Midwife* July–August. 3 (7): 31–3

Marchant, S., Alexander, J., Garcia J., *et al.* (1999) A survey of women's experiences of vaginal loss from 24 hours to three months after childbirth (the BliPP study). *Midwifery* 15 (2): 72–81

Mead, M. (1996) The diagnosis of foetal distress: a challenge to midwives. *Journal of Advanced Nursing* 23: 975–83

Mills, J. E. and Tudehope, D. (2001) Fibreoptic phototherapy for neonatal jaundice. *The Cochrane Library.* Issue 1 Ant. No. CD002060. DOI: 10.1002/14651858.CD.002060

Misuse of Drugs Act (1985). HMSO, London

Mitchell, T. (1995) *The Crimson File. CTGs – Guidance for Interpretation.* West Midlands Perinatal Audit. Solihull Hospital

Mitchell, M. and Doyle, M. (2002) Evaluating a new course in postnatal care. *British Journal of Midwifery* 10 (12): 746–50

Mitchell, E. A., Williams, S. M. and Taylor, B. J. (1999) Use of duvets and the risk of sudden infant death syndrome. *Archives of Diseases in Childhood* August. 81 (2): 117–19

Morley, A. (2004) Pre-eclampsia: pathophysiology and its management. *British Journal of Midwifery* January. 12 (1): 30–1, 34–7

Mortimore, V. R. and McNabb, M. (1998) A six year retrospective analysis of shoulder dystocia and delivery of the shoulders. *Midwifery* 14: 162–73

Moyzakitis, W. (2004) Exploring women's descriptions of distress and/or trauma in childbirth from a feminist perspective. *Evidence Based Midwifery* 2 (1): 8–14

Naughten, F. (2005) The heel prick: how efficient is common practice? *Midwives* 8 (3): 112–14

Nelson, K. B., Dambrisua, L. M., Ting T. Y., *et al.* (1996) Uncertain value of electronic fetal monitoring in predicting cerebral palsy. *The New England Journal of Medicine* 7th March. 334 (10): 613–18

Newton, C. and Champion, P. (1997) Oral intake in labour: Nottingham's policy formulated and audited. *British Journal of Midwifery* July. 5 (7): 418–22

NICE (National Institute for Clinical Excellence) (2001a) *The Use of Electronic Fetal Monitoring. Inherited Clinical Guideline C.* National Institute for Clinical Excellence

NICE (National Institute for Clinical Excellence) (2001b) *Induction of Labour. Inherited Clinical Guideline D.* National Institute for Clinical Excellence

NICE (National Institute for Clinical Excellence) (2003) *Antenatal Care: Routine Care for the Healthy Pregnant Woman. Clinical Guideline.* National Institute for Clinical Excellence

Nicholas, H. (1998) Gonorrhoea: symptoms and treatment. *Nursing Times* 25th February. 94 (8): 52–4

Nikodem, V. C., Danziger, D., Gebka, N., *et al.* (1993) Do cabbage leaves prevent breast engorgement? A randomised, controlled study. *Birth* June. 20 (2): 61–4

NMC (2002) (Nurses and Midwives Council) *Guidelines for the Administration of Medicines.* Nurses and Midwives Council, London

NMC (2004a) (Nurses and Midwives Council) *The NMC Code of Professional Conduct: Standards for Conduct, Performance and Ethics.* Nurses and Midwives Council, London

NMC (2004b) (Nurses and Midwives Council) *Midwives' Rules and Standards.* Nurses and Midwives Council, London

Nocon, J. J., McKenzie, D. K., Thomas, L. J., *et al.* (1993) Shoulder dystocia: an analysis of risks and obstetric maneuvers. *American Journal of Obstetrics and Gynaecology* June. 168 (6): 1732–9. Abstract in: *MIDIRS Midwifery Digest* (1993) December. 3 (4): 427

Nolan, M. (1998) Teenage pregnancy: a challenge for the Government and nation. *Maternity Action* July/August/September. 81: 6–8

Norman, C. (1995) Does nature know best? Background and mechanisms of natural family planning. *Midwives* March. 108 (1284): 85–8

North, R. A., Taylor, R. S. and Schellenberg, J. C. (1999) Evaluation of a definition of pre-eclampsia *British Journal of Obstetrics and Gynaecology* August. 106 (8): 767–73

Nutt, J. (1997) HELLP syndrome. *British Journal of Midwifery* January. 5 (1): 8–11

Olah, K. S. (1994) Subcuticular perineal repair using a new, continuous technique. *British Journal of Midwifery* February. 2 (2): 67–71

Olsen, O. (1999) Expected date of delivery. *British Journal of Obstetrics and Gynaecology* September. 106 (9): 1000

Page, L. (1993) Changing Childbirth. *MIDIRS Midwifery Digest* December. 3 (4): 385–7

Parnell, C., Langhoff-Ross, J., Iverson, R., *et al.* (1993) Pushing method in the expulsive phase of labour: a randomised trial. *Acta Obstetrica et Gynaecologica Scandinavica* January. 72 (1): 31–5. Abstract in *MIDIRS Midwifery Digest* June 1993. 3 (2): 188–9

Parsons, C. (1997) The importance of a healthy pelvic floor. *Modern Midwife* January. 7 (1): 10–14

Percival, P. (2003) Chapter 46: Jaundice and infection. In *Myles Textbook for Midwives* 14th edition (eds D. M. Fraser and M. A. Cooper). Churchill Livingstone, Edinburgh

Prabulos, A. M. and Philipson, E. H. (1998) Umbilical cord prolapse: is the time from diagnosis to delivery critical? *Journal of Reproductive Medicine* February. 43 (2): 129–32. Abstract in: *MIDIRS Midwifery Digest* September 1998. 8 (3): 342

Premkumar, G. (2005) Perineal trauma: reducing associated postnatal maternal morbidity. *Midwives* January. 8 (1): 30–2

Pritchard, M. A., Beller, E. M. and Norton, B. (2005) Skin exposure during conventional phototherapy in preterm infants: a randomized controlled trial. *NNIC* March–April. 18 (2): 25–7

Rantakallio, P., Laara, E. and Koiranen, M. (1995) A 28 year follow up of mortality among women who smoked during pregnancy. *British Medical Journal* 19th August. 311: 477–80

Redfern, J. and Chambers, J. (1996) Itching in pregnancy? Midwives must be alert. *Midwives* February. 109 (1297): 36–7

Roberts, A. (1996) Endocrine function of the pancreas. *Nursing Times* 92 (37): 38–40

Roberts, J. M. (1999) Is oxidative stress the link in the two-stage model of pre-eclampsia? *The Lancet* 4th September. 354: 788–9

Robinson, J. (1998) Dying for sex? Intercourse in the puerperium. *British Journal of Midwifery* November. 6 (11): 732–3

Robinson, J. (1999) When delivery is torture – postnatal PTSD. *British Journal of Midwifery* November. 7 (11): 684

Ruby, C. (1997) Vitamin K prophylaxis: a historical perspective. *MIDIRS Midwifery Digest* September. 7 (30): 362–4

Ruby, C. (1998) Commentary on DoH guidelines on vitamin K for newborn babies. *MIDIRS Midwifery Digest* September. 8 (3): 350–1

Saunders, D. (1997) CESDI: a review. *Modern Midwife* April. 7 (4): 15–19

Schott, J (2002a) Parent education: should it include relaxation and breathing? *Practising Midwife* February. 5 (2): 35–7

Schott, J. (2002b) Preparing for life after birth. *Practising Midwife* June. 5 (6): 37–9

Schott, J. and Henley, A. (1996) Names, notes and records: a cultural perspective. *British Journal of Midwifery* September. 4 (9): 458–61

Severine, J. E. and McKenzie, N. E. (1999) Advances in temperature monitoring: a far cry from 'shake and take'. *Nursing* May. 29 (5): supplement

Shakespeare, D. (2004) Exploring midwives' attitudes to teenage pregnancy. *British Journal of Midwifery* May. 12 (5): 320–6, 329

Sharp, D. A. (1997) Restriction of oral intake for women in labour. *British Journal of Midwifery* July. 5 (7): 408–12

Sheridan, V. (1999) Skin-to-skin contact immediately after birth. *The Practising Midwife* October. 2 (8): 23–8

Sibai, B. M. (2004a) Diagnosis, controversies and management of the syndrome of hemolysis, elevated liver enzymes, and low platelet count. *Obstetrics and Gynecology* May. 103 (5 part 1): 981–91

Sibai, B. M. (2004b) Magnesium sulphate prophylaxis in pre-eclampsia: lessons learned from recent trials. *American Journal of Obstetrics and Gynecology* June. 190 (6): 1520–6

Sibai, B. M. (2005) Diagnosis, prevention and management of eclampsia. *Obstetrics and Gynecology* February. 105 (2): 402–10

Sidebotham, M. (1998) CESDI: the fifth annual report. *British Journal of Midwifery* November. 6 (11): 692–4

Silverstone, T. (1997) Barrier contraceptives. Condoms: still the most popular contraceptive. *Professional Care of Mother and Child* 7 (4): 108–10

Simmons, D. (1997) Persistently poor pregnancy outcomes in women with insulin dependent diabetes. *British Medical Journal* 2nd August. 315: 263–4

Smaill, F. (2001) Antibiotics for asymptomatic bacteriuria in pregnancy. *The Cochrane Database of Systematic Reviews* Issue 2 Art. No. CD000490. DOI:10.1002/14651858. CD000490

Smith, L. (1998) Bacterial vaginosis. *Nursing Times* 11th February 94 (6): 50–1

Squire, C. (2002) Chapter 9: Shoulder dystocia and umbilical cord prolapse. In *Emergencies Around Childbirth: A Handbook for Midwives* (ed. M. Boyle). Radcliffe Medical Press, Abingdon, Oxon.

Steen, M. (1998) Perineal trauma: how do we evaluate its severity? *MIDIRS Midwifery Digest* June. 8 (2): 228–30

Steen, M. (1999) The FemPad, a breakthrough in perineal pain relief. *British Journal of Midwifery* April. 7 (4): 222, 224

Steen, M. and Cooper, K. (1998) Cold therapy and perineal wounds: too cool or not too cool? *British Journal of Midwifery* September. 6 (9): 572–9

Steer, P. J. (1999) The definition of pre-eclampsia. *British Journal of Obstetrics and Gynaecology* August. 106 (8): 753–5

Stevens, T. P., Blennow, M. and Soll, R. F. (2005) Early surfactant administration with brief ventilation vs selective surfactant and continued mechanical ventilation for preterm infants with or at risk for respiratory distress syndrome. *The Cochrane Library* (Oxford) (3) (ID#CD003063)

Stuart, C. C. (2003) Invasive actions in labour: Where have all the 'old tricks' gone? In *Midwifery Best Practice* (ed. S. Wickham). Books for Midwives Press, Edinburgh

Sultan, A. H. (1997) Anal incontinence after childbirth. *Current Opinion in Obstetrics and Gynaecology* October. 9 (5): 320–4. Extracts in *MIDIRS Midwifery Digest* June 1998. 8 (2): 231–3

Sumner, V. (2002) Underinformed on puerperal psychosis, antenatal and postnatal depression: where are we now and where should we be going? *Community Practitioner* August. 75 (8): 316

Symons, A. (1998) Is using CTG defensive? *British Journal of Midwifery* September. 6 (9): 568–70

Thompson, J. (2004) Health problems of women following childbirth: part one. *Community Practitioner* 77 (7): 267

Thomson, A. M. (1993a) If you are pregnant and smoke, admission to hospital may damage your baby's health. *Journal of Clinical Nursing* 2: 111–19

Thomson, A. M. (1993b) Pushing Technique in the second stage of labour. *Journal of Advanced Nursing* February. 18 (2): 171–7

Thomson, A. M. (1995) Maternal behaviour during spontaneous and directed pushing in the second stage of labour. *Journal of Advanced Nursing* 22: 1027–34

Tiran, D. and Mack, S. (eds) (1995) *Complementary Therapies for Pregnancy and Childbirth.* Baillière Tindall, London

Tolliss, D. (1995) Who was . . . Down? *Nursing Times* 1st Feb. 91 (5): 61

Torrance, C. and Semple, M. (1998a) Recording temperature – 1. Practical procedures for nurses 6.1. *Nursing Times* 14th January. 94 (2): no page nos.

Torrance, C. and Semple, M. (1998b) Recording temperature – 2. Practical procedures for nurses 6.2. *Nursing Times* 21st January. 94 (3): no page nos.

Turner, A. (1999a) How to cope with haemorrhoids during pregnancy. *British Journal of Midwifery* November. 7 (11): 722

Turner, E. (1999b) Gestational diabetes: pathophysiology and personal experiences. *Journal of Diabetes Nursing* 3 (3): 90–3

Ursell, B. (2005) Management of iron deficiency in pregnancy. *Midwives* 8 (2): 78–9

Urwin, J. (1995) Emergency contraception. *Maternal and Child Health* October: 320, 322, 324

van den Akker, O. B. A., Andre, J., Lees, S. and Murphy, T. (1999) Adolescent sexual behaviour and knowledge. *British Journal of Midwifery* December. 7 (12): 765–9

Ventolini, G., Samlowski, R. and Hood, D. L. (2004) Placental findings in low-risk, singleton, term pregnancies after uncomplicated deliveries. *American Journal of Perinatology* August. 21 (6): 325–8

Vincent, M. (2003) Progress in a pocket. *Midwives* February. 6 (2): 82–4

Walker, J. and Pollard, L. (1995) Parent education for Asian mothers. *Modern Midwife.* September: 22–3

Walmsley, K. (2000) Managing the OP labours . . . occipito posterior position. *MIDIRS Midwifery Digest* November. 10 (1): 61–2

Walsh, D. (1998) Electronic fetal heart monitoring: revisited and reappraised. *British Journal of Midwifery* June. 6 (6): 400–3

Walton, I. and Hamilton, M. (1995) *Midwives and Changing Childbirth.* Books for Midwives Press, Hale, Cheshire

Ward, C. and Mitchell, A. (2004) The experience of early motherhood – implications for care. *Evidence Based Midwifery* 2 (1): 15–19

Warren, C. (2003) Why should I do vaginal examinations? In *Midwifery Best Practice* (ed. S. Wickham). Books for Midwives Press, Edinburgh

Warwick, K. (1996) Diagnosis and treatment for cholestasis in pregnancy. *Midwives* February. 109 (1297): 37–8

Waterhouse, C. (1994) Midwifery care for orthodox Jewish women. *Modern Midwife* September: 11–14

Waters, J. (1996) Yellow peril. *Nursing Times* 19th June. 92 (25): 16–17

Watkins, P. J. (1998) Pregnancy in diabetes: success or failure? *Diabetic Medicine* 15: 95

Waugh, P. (2000) Culture and family planning. *Practice Nursing* 11 (2): 24–7

Webb, P. (1992) *Homeopathy for Midwives (and pregnant women)*. British Homeopathic Society, London

Webster, J., Pritchard, M. A., Creedy, D. and East, C. (2003) A simplified predictive index for the detection of women at risk for postnatal depression. *Birth* 30 (2): 101–8

West, J. and Topping, A. (2000) Breast-feeding policies: are they used in practice? *British Journal of Midwifery* 8 (1): 36–40

Weston, A. (1998a) Warts and all. *Nursing Times* 21st January. 94 (3): 26–8

Weston, A. (1998b) Striking back at syphilis. *Nursing Times* 21st January. 94 (3): 30–2

Whitton, H. (1995) Infant resuscitation in parenthood education. *Health Visitor* November. 68 (11): 454–5

Williamson, A., Mullet, J., Bunting, M. and Eason, J. (2005) Neonatal examination: are midwives clinically effective? *Midwives* 8 (3): 116–18

Winterton Report (1992) *Parliamentary Select Committee on Health. Second Report on the Maternity Services*. Vol. 2. HMSO, London

Wisborg, K., Kesmodel, U., Henriksen, T. B., *et al.* (2001) Exposure to tobacco smoke in utero and the risk of stillbirth and death in the first year of life. *American Journal of Epidemiology* 154 (4): 322–7

Wray, J. and Jackson-Baker, A. (2000) Anti-D immunoglobulin and antenatal prophylaxis. *Midwives* February. 3 (2): 59–6

Wright, T. (1998) Genital warts: their aetiology and treatment. *Nursing Times* 18th February. 94 (7): 52–4

Young, M. (1997) Problems affecting Asian women with diabetes. *Professional Nurse* May. 12 (8): 565–7

Young, S. and Fleming, P. (1999) Sudden infant death: reducing the risk. *Community Practitioner.* July. 72 (7): 201–4

Zaidi, F. (1994) The maternity care of Muslim women. *Modern Midwife* March: 8–10